SUCCESSFUL

TAEKWON-DO

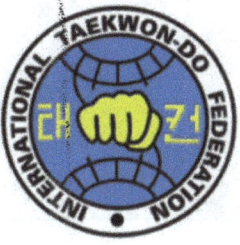

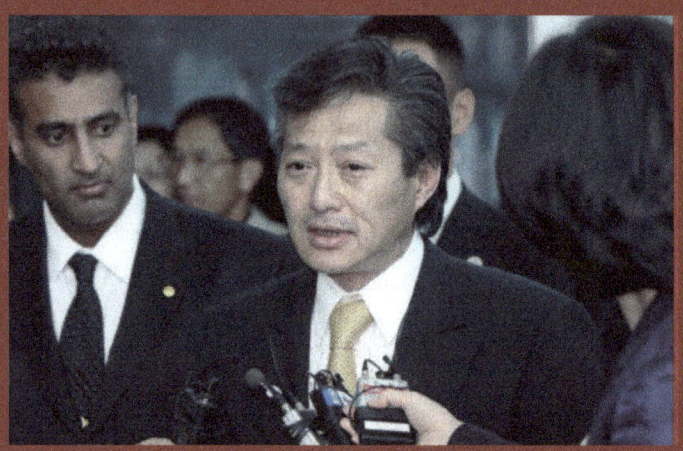

This book is warmly dedicated to Grandmaster Choi Jung Hwa, for his endless dedication, diligence and involvement in modern Taekwon-Do.

With all our respect and admiration.

SUCCESSFUL TAEKWON-DO

Volume One
FUNDAMENTALS

Paul van Beersum
Willem Jansen

CheckPoint Press

Copyright © 2013 by Paul van Beersum & Willem Jansen.

All rights reserved. Printed in the United Kingdom and/or the USA / Australia / Canada / Germany / Brazil. No part of this publication may be reproduced, stored in a retrieval system, or transmitted, in any form or by any means, digital, electronic, mechanical, photocopying, recording, or otherwise, without the prior written permission of the publisher or the author(s) [as per CheckPoint Press contract terms]; except in the case of reviewers who may quote brief passages in a review.

Successful Taekwon-Do: Vol I - Fundamentals

ISBN-13: 978-1-906628-58-1 (2nd Edition 2013)

Published by CheckPoint Press, Ireland

www.checkpointpress.com

(1st edition entitled 'Taekwon-Do: The Way to Success Vol I - Fundamentals')

TABLE OF CONTENTS

Preface	9
Recommendations	10
Introduction	12
PART I – BOOK OF THEORY	13
CHAPTER 1. BASIC PRINCIPLES	15
1.1 The Dojang or practice space	15
Dojang etiquette	15
Interior of the Dojang	16
1.2 Colors of the belts	17
Holder of the 1st dan	17
1.3 Greeting procedure	18
Bow	18
1.4 Instruction	20
CHAPTER 2. HISTORY AND ORGANIZATION OF TAEKWON-DO	21
2.1 Brief history of martial arts	22
2.2 History of Taekwon-Do	22
Korea and its history of martial arts	22
Development of Taekwon-Do	25
Basic principles of Taekwon-Do movements according to the founder	26
WTF and ITF	27
ITF Royal Dutch	27
Taegeukgi	28
CHAPTER 3. TAEKWON-DO, A WAY OF LIFE	33
3.1 A closer look at Taekwon-Do	33
Tenets	34
3.2 The pedagogical value of Taekwon-Do	36
CHAPTER 4. PHYSICAL ASPECTS OF TAEKWON-DO	39
4.1 Basic motor skills	39
Strength and endurance	39
Speed	40
Flexibility	41
4.2 Warming up and cooling down	41
4.3 Stretching	41
Static method	43
Feet and ankle stretches	44
Front and back leg stretches	44
Inner thigh stretches	47

Lower back, hip joint and pelvic floor stretches	47
Back stretches	48
Stomach and chest stretches	49
Arm, elbow, and shoulder girdle stretches	51
Ballistic method	51
Front and back leg stretches	51
(Isometric) partner exercises	51
Front and back leg stretches	51
Inner thigh stretches	52
Breathing and counting	52
4.4 Nutrition	53

Chapter 5. Mental Aspects of Taekwon-Do 57
5.1 Chi	57
5.2 Chakras	58
5.3 Meridians	58
5.4 Vital parts (*Kupso*)	58
5.5 Meditation (*Mong nyom*)	61
5.6 Kihap	61

Chapter 6. Practical Taekwon-Do 63
6.1 Training materials	63
Dallyon Joo (forging post)	64
Speedball	64
Hand mitt	64
Punching bag	64
Mirror	65
Alternatives	65
6.2 Classifications of techniques	65
Arrangement of techniques into categories	66
Striking surfaces	70
Remaining striking surfaces	76
6.3 Stances (*Sogi*)	76
Attention stance (*Charyot Sogi*)	76
Parallel stance (*Narani Sogi*)	76
Closed stance (*Moa Sogi*)	77
Walking stance (*Gunnun Sogi*)	77
Low stance (*Nachuo Sogi*)	78
L-stance (*Niunja Sogi*)	78
Fixed stance (*Gojung Sogi*)	79
Sitting stance (*Annun Sogi*)	80
X-stance (*Kyocha Sogi*)	80
Rear foot stance (*Dwitbal Sogi*)	81
Vertical stance (*Soojik Sogi*)	82
Bending ready stance (*Guburyo Junbi Sogi*)	82
6.4 Starting point	84

Starting point with crossed arms	84
Starting point with both arms	87
Separate starting point	88
Hip use	89
Turning movement	89
Tightening and relaxing	89
Countermovement	89
6.5 Strength development and starting points in Taekwon-Do movements	89
Strength factors	90
Reaction force	90
Concentration	90
Balance	90
Mass	91
Breathing	91
Speed	92
Additional elements	93
Interception and reactive power	94
Turning	94
Relaxation – tension	94
Muscular tension	94
Snap movement	94
Sine wave motion	95
Flow	95
The art of thinking without thinking	95
6.6 Sparring	95
Intercepting the opponent's attack	98
Counterattacking during the opponent's attack	98
Counterattack	98
Making combinations	98
Making feints	98
Applying pressure	98
6.7 Flying techniques	99
Tips	100
Special techniques	100
6.8 Break tests up to the 1st dan	108
Power break tests	108
Precision and control break tests	110
Correct execution	111
Hardening the body parts	111
Correct preparation	111
Mental relaxation and balance	111
Epilogue	115
Acknowledgements	117
About the authors	119

Appendix 1. Glossary of Korean words and definitions   121
Appendix 2. General overview of definitions   125
Appendix 3. Interpretation of the emblem of Taekwon-Do Academie Gelderland   129
Appendix 4. Recommended and consulted literature   131
Appendix 5. Useful addresses and websites   133
Appendix 6. ITF Pattern Instruction Cards   134

TABLE OF CONTENTS PART 2   135

PREFACE

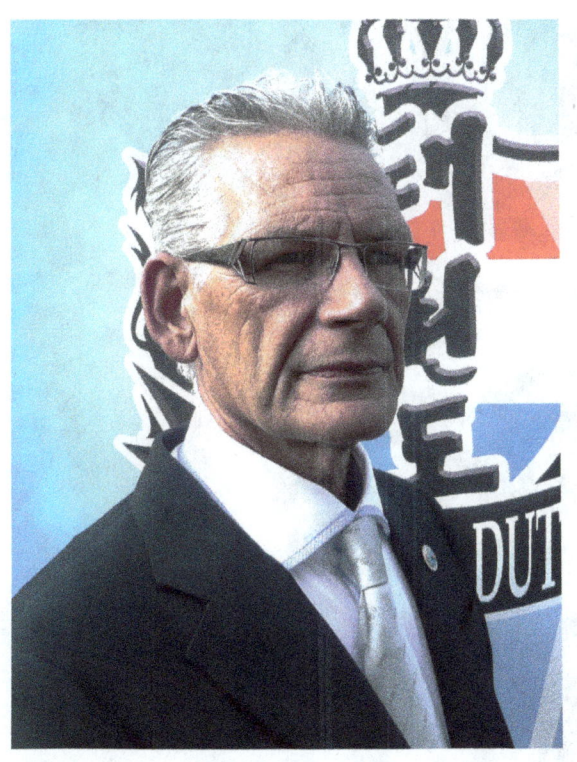

Over the last few years, Taekwon-Do – a martial art with a long history and tradition – has become known in large parts of the world. Developed in Korea as an art of defense, Taekwon-Do has always focused on both spiritual and physical aspects.

Certain well-kept secrets have gradually been revealed from 1850 and on. The founder of Taekwon-Do is General Choi Hong Hi (9th dan), former President of the International Taekwon-Do Federation (ITF). In Korea Choi Hong Hi learned T'aekkyŏn, a Korean martial art which existed of varied leg techniques and had been locally known for over 1300 years. In Japan Choi Hong Hi learned Karate. Consequently, somewhere around the 1950s a synthesis of T'aekkyŏn and Karate came into existence: Taekwon-Do. In the 1960s, Kwon Moo Gun was the first Korean to introduce Taekwon-Do in the Netherlands. The country became even more acquainted with Taekwon-Do due to the many impressive demonstrations by Park Jong Soo.

This great interest in Taekwon-Do requires expert literature. Initiators Paul van Beersum and Willem Jansen have taken the time to write down all information on Taekwon-Do in great detail. Due to their enthusiasm, drive, and urge for perfection they have managed to develop a valuable book for every Taekwon-Do enthusiast. In part because of the excellent technical skills that both gentlemen possess, this book has become interesting and instructive, describing all aspects of Taekwon-Do. This book is a valuable contribution to the further development of Taekwon-Do.

MASTER STEVE ZONDAG, 7TH DAN
– VICE-PRESIDENT ITF ROYAL DUTCH
– PRESIDENT DAN RANKING COMMITTEE
ITF ROYAL DUTCH
– MEMBER OF THE ITF PROMOTIONS COMMITTEE

RECOMMENDATIONS

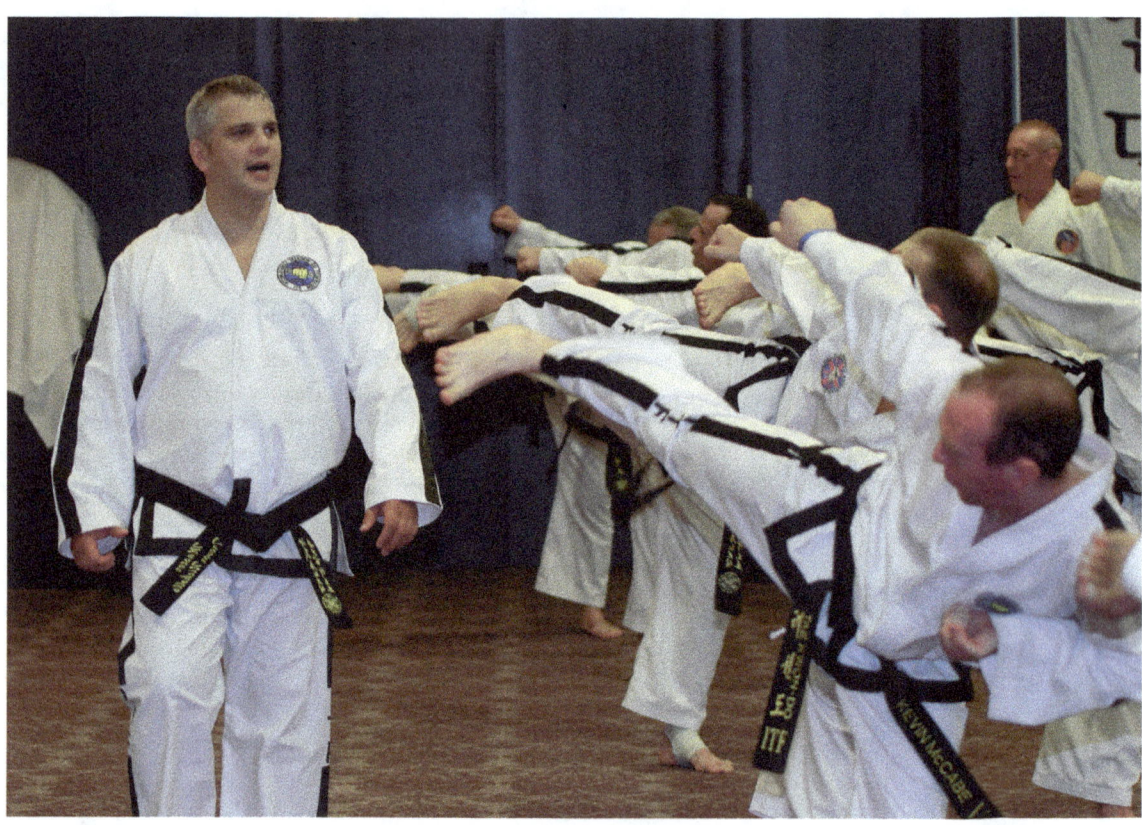

'I congratulate Paul van Beersum and Willem Jansen on the research and diligence invested to produce a useful tool for Taekwon-Do students which complements the theory, explanation and history taught in the Dojang. It is a reflection of the authors' dedication to the art of Taekwon-Do. I hope it will support and encourage Taekwon-Do students in their personal development.'

MASTER TREVOR NICHOLLS 8TH DEGREE
SECRETARY-GENERAL INTERNATIONAL TAEKWON-DO FEDERATION

Tao gives birth to them
Tê keeps them alive
The material world gives them shape
The circumstances complete them

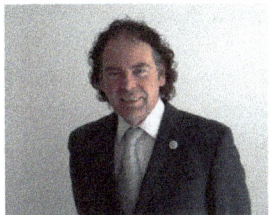

If you are seriously considering practicing Taekwon-Do, first of all it is important to find a good school with a well-trained instructor that is a member of a recognized national and international organization. Furthermore, it is significant to devote a decent amount of time and effort to (self-)study. To help you with this last aspect I highly recommend this book. During the forty-one years I have been practicing Taekwon-Do, teaching at my academy, and have been partially responsible for teachers' education programs for the ITF Royal Dutch, I have studied a great amount of literature on self-defense, including Taekwon-Do.

In my opinion, the book that lies in front of you is a unique one. As an addition to lessons from your instructor, this book is a valuable contribution in acquiring the essential knowledge, skills, and attitude needed to obtain the first dan-degree in ITF Taekwon-Do. Also, it offers a description of the techniques, describes a number of introductory motor skills, and pays attention to nutrition and the educational structure of a lesson. For these reasons the book is useful for those who practice a different martial art as well. It is also a good guideline for teachers in practical education that are interested in expanding their self-defense curriculum with Taekwon-Do. I am thinking of instructors and teachers at a Education Institute, the Central Institutes for the Education of Sports Instructors, an Academy for Physical Education or a vocational training at the police or Ministry of Defense.

The four sentences in italics that can be found above this text certainly apply to the two authors. I have known both authors since they were young, and have had the pleasure of coaching them as their teacher and examiner within the teacher training program at the Teacher Training College Committee (TTCC), as they developed from assistant-teacher to head teacher. What has struck me about these two Taekwon-Doins throughout the years is their excellent technical fluency, their perseverance, their passion for our martial art, their positive characters, the respect they have for others, and their pedagogical and didactic skills. These qualities have led to the fact that they have obtained a pedagogical first degree practical education on an academic level (ALO) and their qualities assure that the lessons within their Taekwon-Do Academie Gelderland are of a guaranteed quality. The combination of these qualities and the fact that, after much study, they have written this book, makes these two gentlemen unique teachers that everyone would want on their team. I am among the lucky ones, since they were willing to join my educational team at the Teacher Training College Committee in 2010. The Teacher Training College Committee has a long history, is unique in the field of Taekwon-Do education and is open to every Taekwon-Do student who is interested in becoming an assistant-instructor, instructor, or chief instructor. Whit pedagogical, psychological and didactical qualities. A (short term) plan is to start our teacher training programs on an international level, in cooperation with the ITF world organization of grandmaster Choi Jung Hwa (son of General Choi Hong Hi, the founder of Taekwon-Do). Because of its qualitative and varied content, this book will become a part of ITF Royal Dutch's subject material as well.

In conclusion, this book will be a significant contribution to the aforementioned target groups. In addition, I hope this book will stimulate Taekwon-Do students with pedagogical, psychological and didactical qualities and/or interests to follow a teacher training program at ITF Royal Dutch. Also, may it inspire already trained instructors to optimize stimulating, good, and safe education.

SABUM HENNIE THIJSSEN BC, M.A. 6TH DAN
– PRESIDENT ITF ROYAL DUTCH
– PRESIDENT TEACHER TRAINING COLLEGE COMMITTEE
– MEMBER OF THE DAN RANKING COMMITTEE ITF ROYAL DUTCH

INTRODUCTION

In front of you lies *Taekwon-Do, the Way to success*. It is a book that explains the basics of Taekwon-Do through writing and illustrations, in a structured and clear manner. Numerous books have been written on martial arts in general, and Taekwon-Do in particular. The authors have read, studied, and are in possession of many of these books.

Still, the authors have chosen to add a new book to the great amount of existing literature. A book that captures the essence of several important works in the field of Taekwon-Do, that makes choices which are illustrated with images. This makes this book *the* core book for every serious student of Taekwon-Do, not in the least for the students of the Taekwon-Do Academy Gelderland (TAG).

References to (other) English or Korean books have partially become redundant, since the more than 750 pictures and illustrations sometimes say more than a thousand words. Moreover, the book takes an important stand for the value of Taekwon-Do.

From the very first introduction to Taekwon-Do, to the exam material for the 1st dan, the black belt; this book offers insights at every level. For the beginning student, this book offers an extensive overview of the history, customs, expectations, and principles of instruction of Taekwon-Do. For the student attempting to acquire the 1st dan, this book is most importantly an exercise book, for the dan rank holder it is a significant reference book, meant to refresh, maintain, and broaden their knowledge.

After reading this book, you will understand that Taekwon-Do is not merely a sport. It is a way of life, a path one chooses when practicing Taekwon-Do. It is a path that, through trial and error, will make the Taekwon-Do student stronger in a physical and mental manner - not only as an athlete but also as a human being. Therefore, for the authors Taekwon-Do does not only mean 'the way of the foot and the fist', but also 'the Way to success'. This is the reason the 'W' in the subtitle is written in caps.

The book is composed as follows. Part I contains basic knowledge, which is why we have named it 'Book of Theory'. Part II mainly consists of practical information for practicing towards obtaining the 1st dan, supported by numerous pictures. This is why Part II is named 'Exercise Book'.

Part I is made up of chapters 1 through 6. In Chapter 1, basic principles are discussed; what it is that characterizes Taekwon-Do, etiquette, and other subjects concerning appearance. Chapter 2 deals with the origins of Taekwon-Do and the current practical organization of this martial art. Chapter 3 discusses Taekwon-Do as a lifestyle and its pedagogical value. Chapter 4 describes the physical aspects of practicing Taekwon-Do; Chapter 5 complements this by discussing the mental aspects. Finally, Chapter 6 reveals a tip of the iceberg concerning the practical part of Taekwon-Do. Technical elements and principles are dealt with in this chapter.

Part II consists of only one chapter. In Chapter 1, tuls, self-defense and partner exercises are extensively discussed. If you leaf through the book, you will see this is the largest part of the book. The wide range of techniques that Taekwon-Do has is discussed, offering inspiration to both the beginning and the advanced student. The authors have added Appendixes with useful additional information for Part I and II.

PART I

BOOK OF THEORY

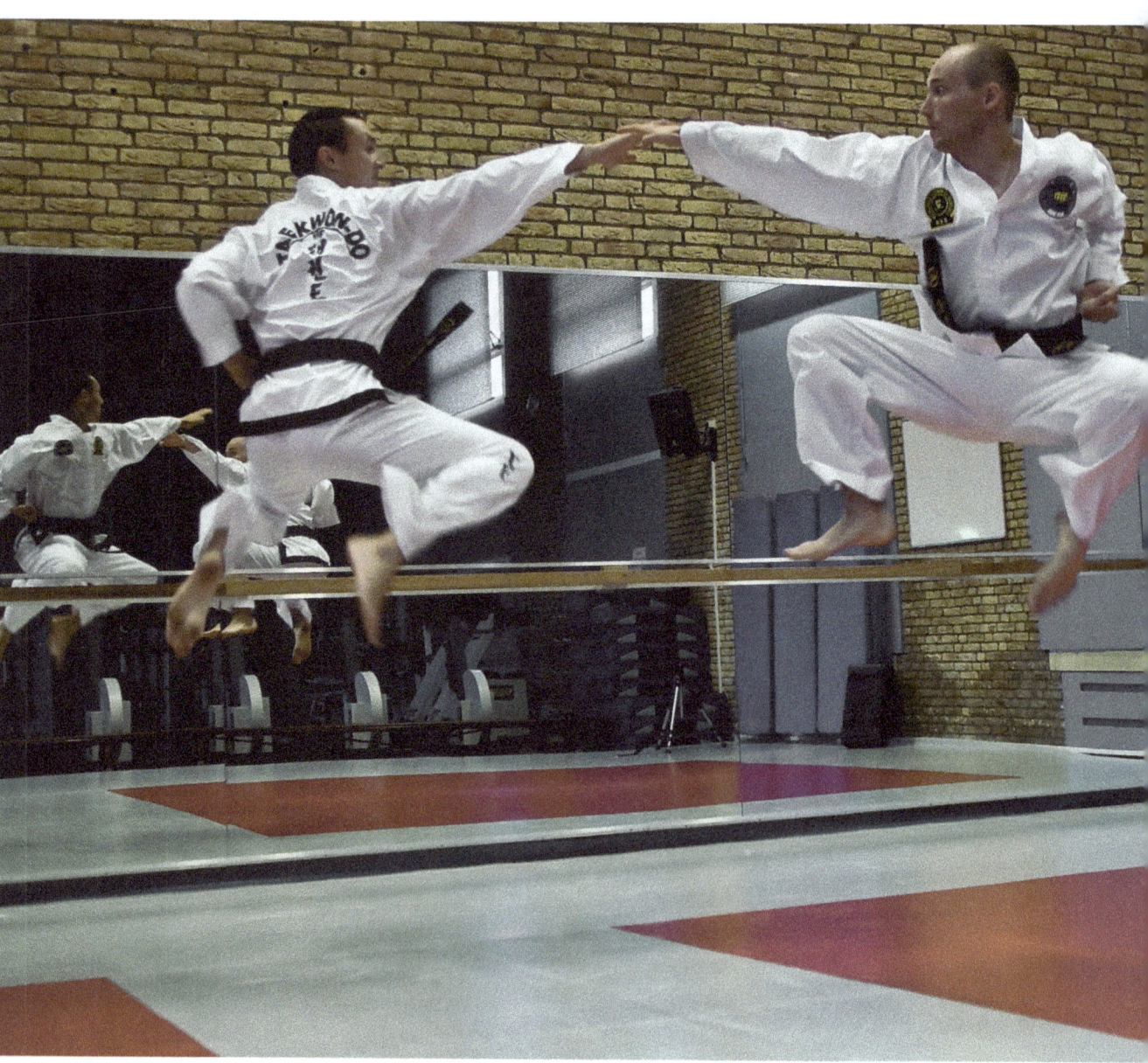

1. BASIC PRINCIPLES

When entering a Dojang for the first time, one is immediately confronted with several eye-catching things. In this chapter, the most important basic elements are discussed in a manner that is easy to comprehend; for the beginning Taekwon-Do student, but also for the advanced student that wants to refresh their knowledge. The way the paragraphs are arranged is similar to the way one first is introduced to Taekwon-Do; when walking into the Dojang for the first time.

1.1. The Dojang or practice space

Literally, Dojang can be translated as 'the place where one learns "the way" (the "Do" in "Taekwon-Do")'. For Koreans, this generally is the place where one learns Korean martial arts. The Dojang is usually a practice space. However, Dojang is also the name that is given to the space in Korean Buddhist temples where one meditates. Therefore, 'the place where one learns "the way"' may refer to the way of Korean martial arts but also to the way of Korean Buddhism. Either way, the Dojang is a serious place which one attends to learn.

There are several rules of conduct attached to the Korean origins of Taekwon-Do. Discipline and the manner of greeting have a particularly significant place in Taekwon-Do. Within the Dojang, but naturally also outside of it, a Taekwon-Doin (one who practices Taekwon-Do) must behave according to the etiquette of Taekwon-Do. The most important goal is to be a human being that is as good as possible, with correct and pure behavior.

The authors at a seminar at the Dojang in Daejeon, South Korea.

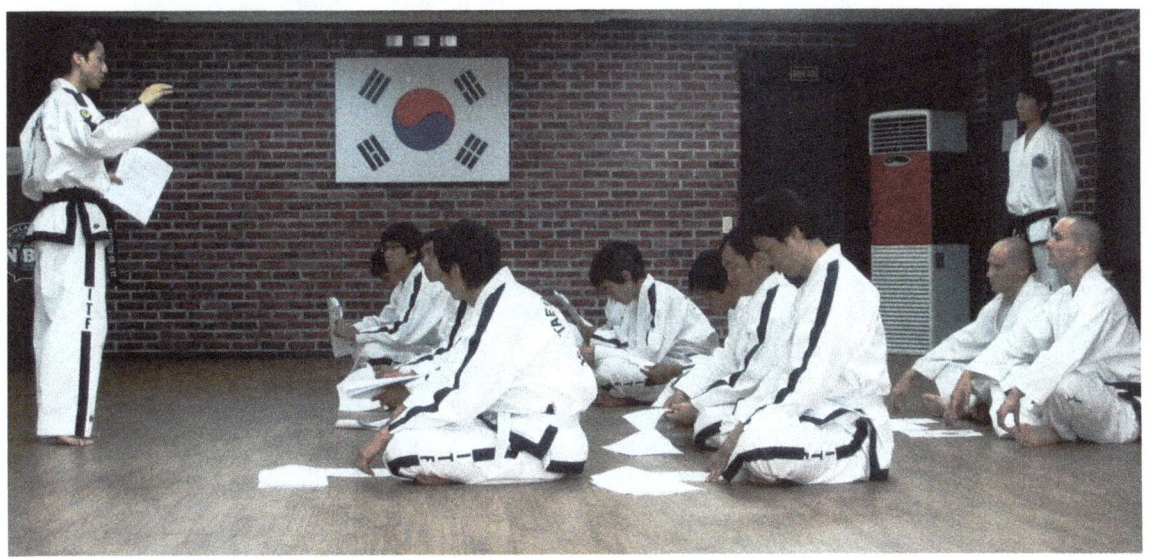

Dojang etiquette

Before entering the Dojang, one needs to:
1. Be well groomed: short nails, clean hands and feet, etc.;
2. Not wear any rings, sharp objects, necklaces, or other jewelry;
3. Keep the *Dobok* (clothing of the way) properly closed, with a belt in the correct color. Also, the belt needs to be properly tied;
4. Take care of possible injuries beforehand, and also during the lesson.

Inside the Dojang:
1. Smoking is prohibited;
2. There is no swearing or useless chatter;
3. Alcohol, sodas, and food are prohibited;
4. Wearing shoes is prohibited;
5. No one is allowed to give instructions without consent from the instructor;
6. No one is allowed to leave the lesson without consent from the instructor;
7. One wears a clean, official *Dobok* during the lesson.

The Taekwon-Do student shows respect to the founder, teacher, and fellow students in the following ways:
1. Before the Dojang is entered, one bows to the Dojang and the ITF[1] flag;
2. One bows to the instructor from an appropriate distance;
3. One greets other students;
4. One bows to the founder and instructor before class starts;
5. One states the oath before class starts;
6. One meditates for one minute after class, sitting with crossed legs;
7. One bows to the instructor and the founder to greet them;
8. One bows to the ITF flag before leaving the Dojang.

The Taekwon-Do oath is:
1. I will honor the Tenets of Taekwon-Do.
2. I will show respect to the instructors and my seniors.
3. I will never abuse Taekwon-Do.
4. I will be a champion in freedom and justice.
5. I will help build a peaceful world.

In Dutch Dojangs these rules are not strictly maintained and spoken out loud. In Korean Dojangs this is the case.

Interior of the Dojang

In the Netherlands, students often practice in a physical education classroom that is rented from a school or the municipality. Some organizations practice in a Dojang that is suited for several martial arts. Often this takes place through a commercial gym.

However, there are certain basic elements that need to be present in a Dojang:
1. A picture of the founder;
2. A flag of the ITF;
3. An instruction board;
4. First aid supplies.

And preferably, but not necessarily:
5. Training materials;
6. Mirror wall;
7. Fall pad.

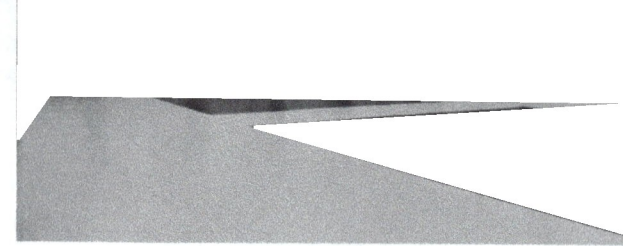

The Dojang in Arnhem, the Netherlands.

---

1. International Taekwon-Do Federation

For the serious Taekwon-Do student who wants to practice at home aside from regular classes, it is not always necessary to have access to a Dojang. It is possible to train in the park, the forest, on the beach, or at another location. Practicing under different circumstances stimulates the development of a Taekwon-Doin. Outdoor training during all seasonal changes is a good example. This way, not only the physical aspects, but also the mental aspects will be trained. This will be discussed later on in the book.

1.2 Colors of the belts

Something that stands out about students of Taekwon-Do is the fact that they wear a colored belt (ti). The colors of the belt symbolize the stage that the student is at at the moment. These stages are:

WHITE
Color of innocence: the beginning student has little knowledge of Taekwon-Do.

YELLOW (8th Kub)
Color of the earth: a plant sprouts and roots itself, such as the student that is acquiring the basics of Taekwon-Do.

GREEN (6th Kub)
Color of the plant, that grows and develops itself. The student is starting to develop itself in the art of Taekwon-Do.

BLUE (4th Kub)
Color of the sky, to which the plant ripens itself. In a similar way, the student develops itself through practice.

RED (2nd Kub)
Color of danger, which warns the student to stay in control, and also warns the adversary to stay away.

BLACK (1st dan)
The opposite of white. It signifies the ripeness and skill in Taekwon-Do.

The Taekwon-Doin is supposed to tie the belt well with a flat knot. The belt is not crossed on the back; the end of the belt has the same length on both sides. Dan rank holders have their name in writing and their rank in Roman numerals embroidered on the belt.

Holder of the 1st dan
A grave misunderstanding is that when one acquires the 1st dan, one is a master or even an expert in Taekwon-Do. The 1st dan is a starting point; Taekwon-Do truly begins after that. Of course, it is also a personal milestone and a nice moment to be allowed to wear the black belt.

In principle, the holder of the black belt has mastered the basics. This means that the fundamental exercises have generally been mastered. There is a great challenge in further developing oneself technically, mentally, and physically.

Between every dan rank there is a 'waiting period', and the higher the student gets, the longer the waiting period is. The waiting period is necessary for physical exercise, but especially for the ripening of the mind.

A Taekwon-Do sabum (instructor) is in possession of the 4th dan. A Taekwon-Do sahyun (master) is in possession of the 7th dan. Acquiring this dan, if ever, requires many years of hard work, submission, loyalty, and dedication. A sharp and serious Taekwon-Do dan rank holder will acknowledge how little he knows when acquiring the 1st dan, and realize that he is far from being an instructor, let alone a master.

The 1st dan rank holder has an important position. Similar to the instructor, the 1st dan rank holder is a role model for students of a lower rank. Moreover, he is also a role model for other 1st dan rank holders. What is his behavior like inside and outside of the Dojang? How does he behave during class? Is he present during every class? In short, the black belt holder has a great responsibility. The 'true' black belt holder is always aware of this responsibility.

1.3 Greeting procedure

In paragraph 1.1 Dojang etiquette has been discussed. Greeting is a part of this. In this paragraph the greeting procedure will be discussed further. In Taekwon-Do, the greeting procedure is an important ritual; it is a part of Taekwon-Do etiquette. It is a ceremony that is based on respect, politeness, friendliness, duty, and courteousness. This is why a correct greeting is highly valued. This is all connected to Asian philosophy, which has had a major influence on the development of Taekwon-Do and the Korean attitude. Therefore, it is important to correctly execute a greeting. In Taekwon-Do, a greeting is generally performed with a standing bow. Below the correct procedure and positions will be mentioned, but even more important are the intention and attitude of the person performing the greeting. It is important not to be rushed or careless, since the greeting has to meet the expectations of the other person involved.

Bow
Before everyone is in position:

Command	Action
• **Charyot**	• Attention stance
• **Changnika nim ke**	• Face towards the founder
• **Kyong Ye**	• Bow

Afterwards (everyone is in position, so Charyot is not necessary):

• **Sabum nim ke**	• Face towards the instructor
• **Kyong Ye**	• Bow

N.B. When an assistant-instructor, master, or grandmaster is teaching the class, the greeting procedure is adapted accordingly.

It is an international custom for the students to reply with 'Taekwon' after the greeting procedure is finished. It is not allowed to answer 'Taekwon' to the founder, since he is not able to reply.

Concerning the execution, the following aspects have to be taken into account:

On the command *Charyot*:

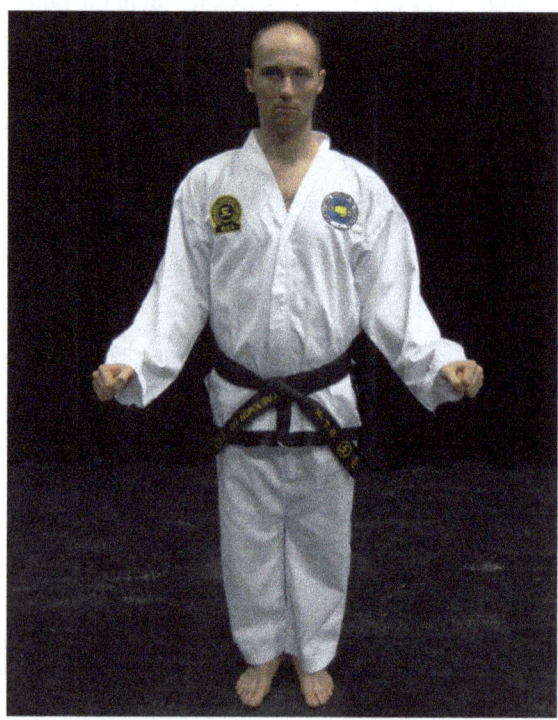

1. Feet are positioned heels together in an angle of 45 degrees.
2. Arms are slightly bent and naturally hanging down; fists are slightly clenched.
3. Eyes and head are facing forward (in the direction to which one bows).

On the command *Kyong Ye*:

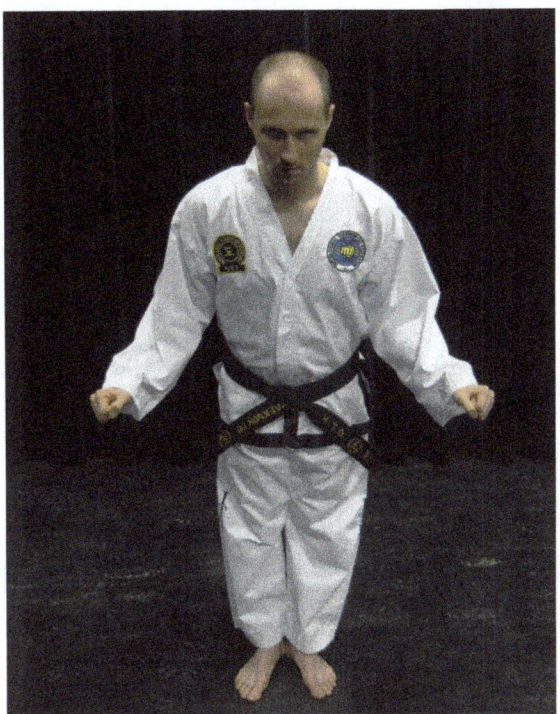

1. Bow upper body 15 degrees forward.
2. Eyes remain focused on instructor/opponent/partner.

Although the greeting procedure is highly valued in Taekwon-Do, this does not mean that the ideal Taekwon-Do student is constantly greeting. This would make the greeting lose its value. Generally, one greets at the beginning and ending of a class, when leaving the Dojang during class, and at the beginning and ending of a partner exercise.

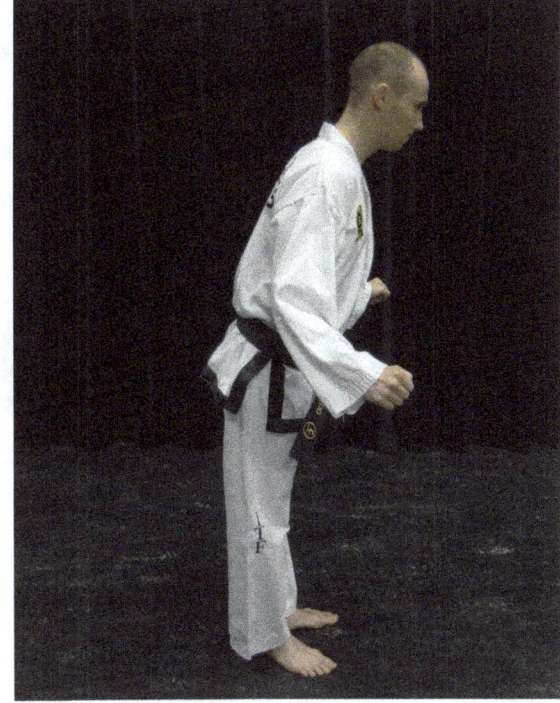

1.4 Instruction

Apart from the interior of the Dojang, the colors of the belts, and the greeting procedure, there is one more thing that catches the eye when entering a Dojang: the (work) atmosphere. The manner of teaching and instructing is different from that of other sports classes or practices. The way of instructing Taekwon-Do contributes to the distinctive etiquette, discipline, the pedagogical and didactical climate and the training methods of this martial art. In general, there are two ways in which the instructor or master teaches the class or student.

1. With command (*Kuryung e machuoso*)
2. Without command (*Kuryong obsi*)

The instruction takes place as follows:

1. The student has their hands against each other on their back, palms open, while slightly pulling the shoulders back and tightening the gluteal muscles. This creates a positive, open attitude which exudes confidence.
2. Upon hearing the command *Charyot*, the student moves into the attention stance. The student makes sure that they are extremely attentive.
3. Upon hearing the command *Kyong Ye*, the student bows towards the instructor and remains in the attention stance.
4. The instructor explains the assignment. The instructor states whether this assignment is with or without command. Then, the instructor gives the command for *Junbi*. At that moment, the student is in *Junbi Jase*; the ready stance.
5. The instructor gives the command *Si Jak* and the student begins with the exercise. If the exercise is with command, the instructor will count out loud. On every count, spoken in Korean, the student will carry out the assignment. The command *Guman* signifies that the student should stop or interrupt the exercise.
6. When the student hears the command Swiyo, they return to the parallel ready stance in a relaxed manner, hands on his back.
7. The command *Hae San* stands for the end of the class. At this time, the student is allowed to walk away or, if appropriate, to remain in the position described at number 1.

Since Taekwon-Do is originally a military martial art, it contains certain stances and procedures that originate from the army. The history of Taekwon-Do will be more extensively discussed in the next chapter. For a clarification of aforementioned commands, forms of address, and names, the authors would like to direct the reader to Appendix 1. This appendix has an extensive overview which can be used to clarify the most common Korean concepts.

2. HISTORY AND ORGANIZATION OF TAEKWON-DO

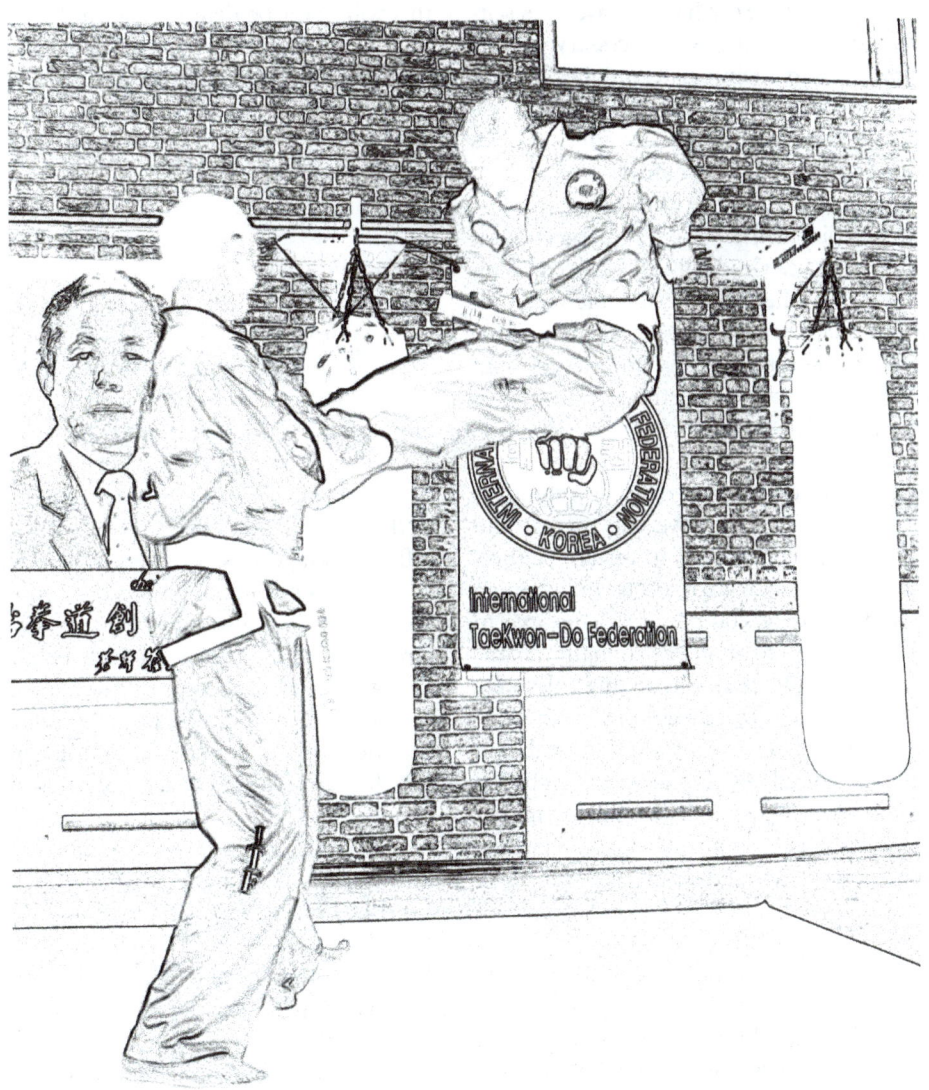

In Chapter 1, the exterior appearance of Taekwon-Do has been discussed. Needless to say, this appearance is not without any foundation. In this chapter, the general history of martial arts and self-defense will be briefly touched upon. In addition, the development of Taekwon-Do will be discussed.

2.1 Brief history of martial arts

Ever since man walked the earth there have been self-defense techniques; fighting was necessary to stay alive. To practice and maintain techniques, people competed among themselves. Practicing self-defense techniques was taken very seriously; after all, lives depended upon it. Aside from natural responses of the human being, other effective techniques were discovered – often coincidentally – by thinking about it or observing animals. Gradually, these techniques were improved until they became suitable weapons. Since every human being is essentially the same, results that were found for invented techniques from the most differing cultures and time periods were often strikingly similar.

As time progressed, certain self-defense techniques developed techniques to improve the mental and physical condition of man. Also, in certain cultures the focus was on pedagogical aspects, maintaining traditions, and forms of competition. The urge to compare one's strength to another's strength is natural for human beings. To be able to do this, rules were developed in order to practice techniques in a competitive atmosphere. This is how it came to be that in one sport it was allowed to grab the opponent by the jacket, whereas in another sport it was only permitted to use the naked body. In other sports, only kicking and punching were allowed. In short, every sport had its own rules.

Also, ways were invented to train potentially dangerous techniques with each other; training with protection. It is not the goal of this book to give a complete description of the enormous amount of fighting techniques and sports that have been developed throughout history, if this is even possible. Not in the least since the descriptions and images that have survived the test of time are often incomplete, and existing knowledge on ancient fighting techniques is very fragmentary. Many of the images were discovered in pyramids and other graves. Even prehistoric cave paintings have been discovered, showing wrestlers and boxers. Some martial artists claim that 'their' sport is the oldest one. However, due to a lack of effective documenting sources in earlier centuries this will never be determined. In the authors' opinion, every martial art is connected to the other – regardless of how old it is – but some branches are more closely connected to each other than others.

2.2 History of Taekwon-Do

Korea and its history of martial arts
Korea has a rich history of several different martial arts. Aside from Taekwon-Do, Korea is the birthplace of *Hapkido, Tang soo do, Kum-do, T'aekkyŏn, Kuk sool won, Hanmudo,* and *Hae dong gumdo,* among others. In this chapter, the early history of Taekwon-Do in particular will be discussed.

In the beginning of our era, Korea consisted of three different kingdoms: Koguryŏ, Paekche, and Silla. During this period, there was a youth organization called *Hwarang*, also known as 'flower boys'. These boys engaged themselves in the arts (singing, dancing, music, and poetry) and wore makeup. It is claimed that these 'flower boys' were above all a militaristic group of young men, but this was definitely not the case. The Hwarang had their own code of honor.

This code consisted of the following points:
1. Be loyal to the king;
2. Obey your parents;
3. Be honorable to your friends;
4. Never retreat from a fight;
5. Kill in a righteous manner.

Although the Hwarang were not directly involved in the development of Taekwon-Do, these five points are

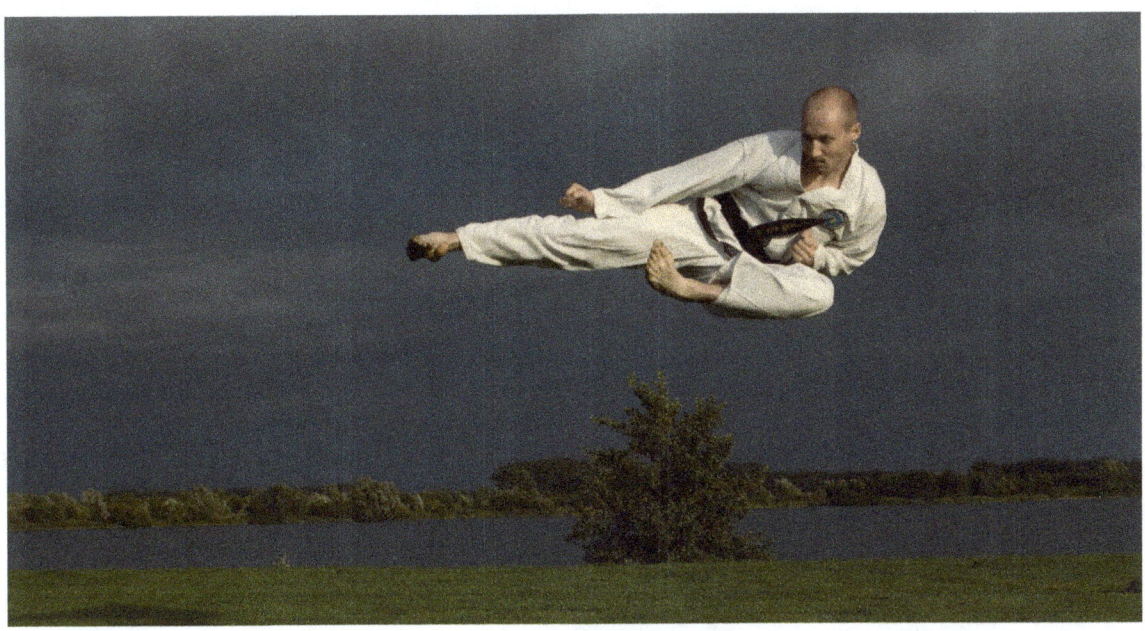

Twimyo Yopcha Jiruqi.

clearly present in the instructional book written by General Choi Hong Hi, founder of modern-day Taekwon-Do. The founder has named pattern 8 (*Hwarang tul*) after this youth organization. Choi Hong Hi wrote his books under the pseudonym Chang Hun, which is why 'his' style of Taekwon-Do is called *Chang-Hun Taekwon-Do*.

During this time period, the most common martial arts in Korea were *Subak* and *T'aekkyŏn*. *Subak* is a martial art that mainly consists of hand strikes. T'aekkyŏn is more of a game-like martial art, which is mainly characterized by its high kick techniques. It is allowed to block the kicks by hand. A misunderstanding about T'aekkyŏn is that it is merely an art from ancient Korea; to this day T'aekkyŏn has many students. General Choi Hong Hi has practiced T'aekkyŏn during his youth.

Throughout the *Koryŏ* dynasty (912-1392) and the Yi dynasty (1392-1910), Korea has endured many foreign attacks and influences. In 1270, Korea was forced to surrender to the Mongolian tribes of the Khan. These Mongolians were known for their flying kick techniques. The Mongolian dynasty was succeeded by the Chinese Ming dynasty. The northern-Chinese (*Shaolin*) martial arts that came into being under the auspices of the Indian monk *Bodhidharma* (also known as Duruma) are characterized by their leg techniques. *Bodhidharma* was also the founder of the Chinese Chan Buddhism, which is better known under its Japanese name: Zen Buddhism. Furthermore, Korea was often harassed by Japanese pirates during these years. All in all, for centuries Korea was influenced by outside cultures.

During the Yi dynasty, militarism in Korea became organized. Korea started taking a more isolated course. Buddhism and the body of thought by philosophers such as *Confucius* and *Lao Zi* became significant religious trends. These religious trends have had a great impact on the Korean way of thinking, opinions, and ethics. Oriental philosophy is therefore interwoven with Korean martial arts.

In times of peace, trade took place with China and Japan. There was much trade in particular with the *Ryūkyū* islands. Okinawa is the main island of this archipelago. Inevitably, fighting techniques have been introduced to Korea through trade. From 1910 until the end of World War II, Korea was occupied by Japan. Korean martial arts were officially prohibited during the occupation. Instead, Japanese martial arts *Kendo* and *Judo* were added to the curriculum. Japan had an enormous influence on Korea during these years. For example, Koreans were forced to join the Japanese army. This caused many Koreans to experience Japanese military training. In hindsight, this time period has been crucial for the development of Taekwon-Do; not only because of the Japanese influences, but also because of the urge for freedom and an own identity that grew among the Korean people.

After World War II, the Korean people occupied themselves with the reconstruction of their country and the search for their 'lost' Korean identity. The Cold War had an impact on this search. At the end of the war, the southern part of the country had been liberated by American troops, whereas the northern part of the country was freed by Russian troops. This had grave consequences for the country; the northern part developed into a communist dictatorial state, whereas the southern part eventually became a democracy. In the 1950s a gruesome war was fought over these ideological differences. Still today, the 38th degree of latitude makes up the border between North and South. The most significant aforementioned facts and events are represented in Figure 2.1.

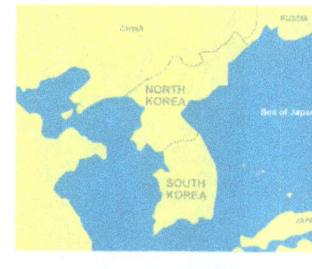

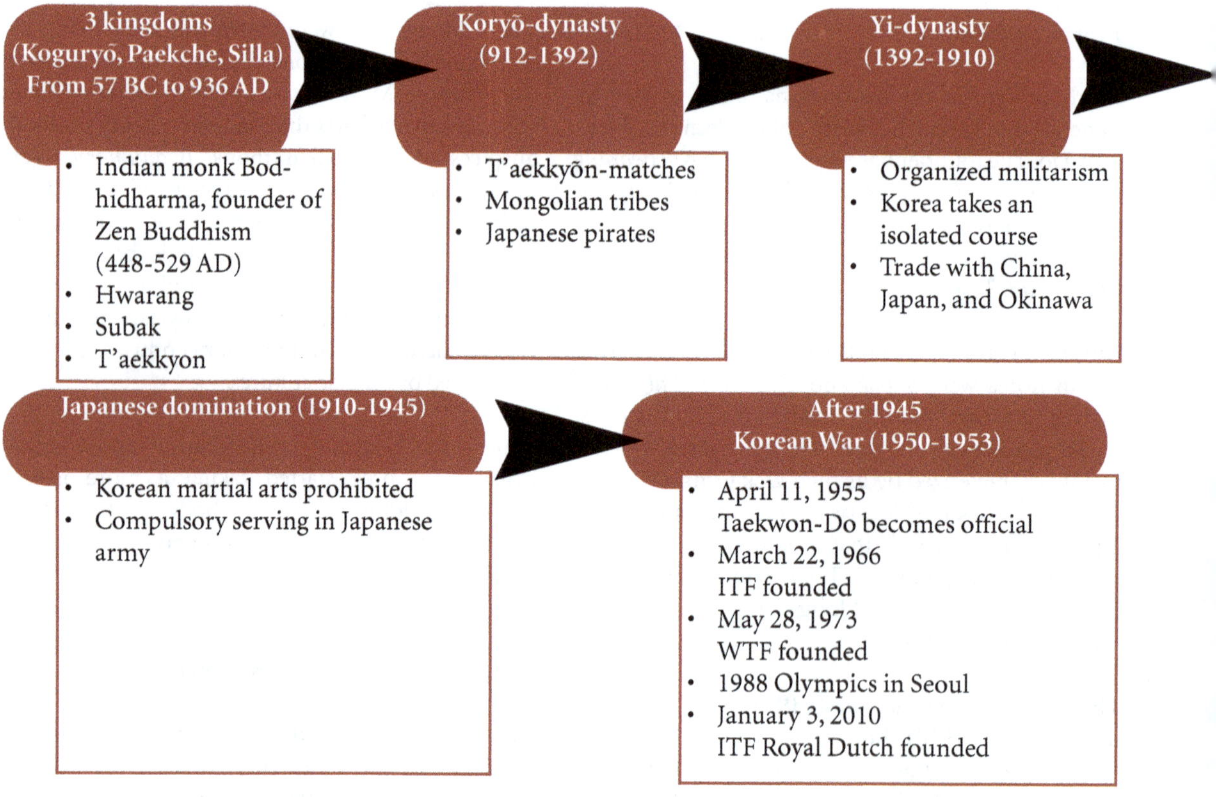

```
3 kingdoms                →  Koryŏ-dynasty      →  Yi-dynasty         →
(Koguryŏ, Paekche, Silla)    (912-1392)            (1392-1910)
From 57 BC to 936 AD
```

- Indian monk Bodhidharma, founder of Zen Buddhism (448-529 AD)
- Hwarang
- Subak
- T'aekkyon

- T'aekkyŏn-matches
- Mongolian tribes
- Japanese pirates

- Organized militarism
- Korea takes an isolated course
- Trade with China, Japan, and Okinawa

Japanese domination (1910-1945) → **After 1945 Korean War (1950-1953)**

- Korean martial arts prohibited
- Compulsory serving in Japanese army

- April 11, 1955 Taekwon-Do becomes official
- March 22, 1966 ITF founded
- May 28, 1973 WTF founded
- 1988 Olympics in Seoul
- January 3, 2010 ITF Royal Dutch founded

Source: Teacher Training College Committee

Figure 2.1 Timeline of Korean martial arts history

Development of Taekwon-Do

General Choi Hong Hi was born on November 9, 1918, during the Japanese occupation, in Hwa Dae, Myong Chun district in North Korea. At the age of 11, Choi was the leader of a freedom movement at his school. For this reason he was expelled from school by the Japanese. His parents then made him study calligraphy. Choi was taught by the famous Han Il-Dong, who was also a master in T'aekkyŏn. Next to the calligraphy lessons Choi learned T'aekkyŏn as well. In 1938, Choi Hong Hi moved to Japan to further his education. There, he was introduced to *Shotokan Karate-Do* and acquired his 2nd dan rank. Also, he was fortunate enough to be taught by Grandmaster Gichin Funakoshi, the father of modern day Karate-Do.

During World War II, Choi Hong Hi had the opportunity to return to Korea, where he founded the national liberation movement. Because of these activities Choi again found himself in trouble with the Japanese, and he was sent to jail. While incarcerated he taught Karate-Do to his fellow inmates. Choi was eventually sentenced to death, but three days before his execution Japan surrendered.

After the liberation of Korea, Choi became second lieutenant in the young Korean Republican Army. He taught his soldiers Karate-Do because of the mental and physical training it required. During this time Taekwon-Do was developed. Choi wanted to develop a unique national martial art. Based on the principles of modern science and Newton's physics in particular, Choi and his associate Nam Tae Hi started to develop a modern martial art. Choi named his style *Chang-Hun*, after the name he took on as a writer. This is why today this style is actually called Chang-Hun Taekwon-Do. Choi founded his own military school and named it *Oh Do Kwan* ('training of my way'). During these days, many *Kwans* were established. In Korean, Kwan means 'house'. On April 11, 1955, a committee gathered together to bring a sense of unity to all these different Kwans. Choi Hong Hi suggested the name *Taekwon-Do* and this was accepted (see Figure 2.2). All the Kwans together now formed Taekwon-Do and focused on the style that was developed by Choi Hong Hi. One Kwan, master Hwang Kee's *Moo Dok Kwan*, did not merge with the other Kwans. This Kwan is now known as the martial art *Tang soo do*.

Figure 2.2 The development of Taekwon-Do from different Kwans

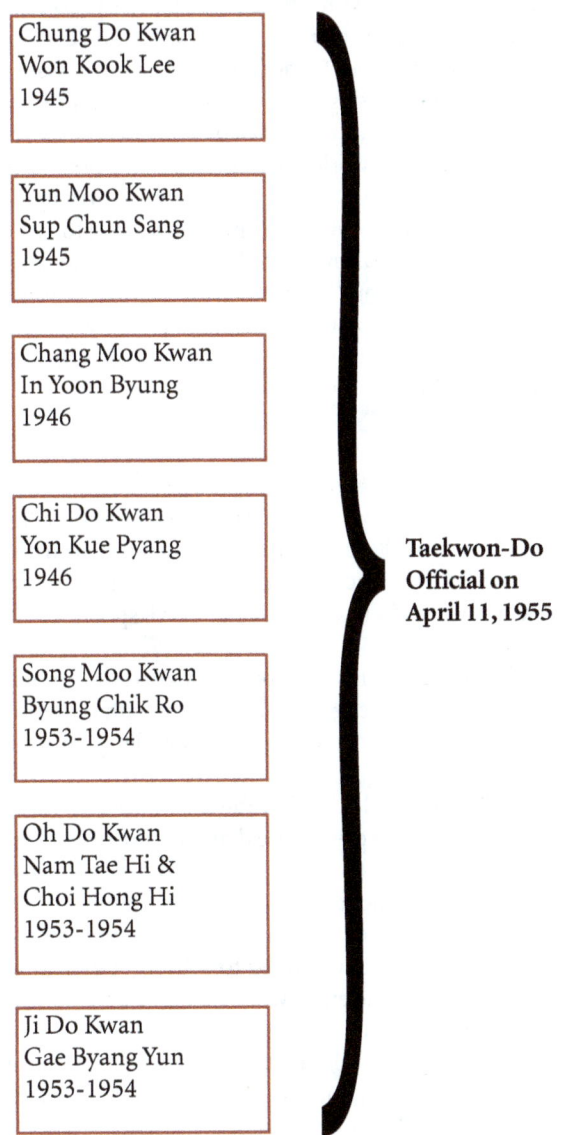

Source: Corcoran, John. *The Martial Arts Companion*. New York: Friedman Group. 1992.

Several years later, in 1961, the Korean Taekwon-Do Association (KTA) was established. Choi Hong Hi became the first president of the KTA. His career in the army also soared and he was eventually appointed general. Choi required all soldiers in the army to learn Taekwon-Do.

In 1966, the International Taekwon-Do Federation came into being, with Choi Hong Hi as its president. Next to constantly being occupied with the development Taekwon-Do, Choi was also the ambassador of Korea during this time. From this moment until the end of his life, Choi traveled to spread Taekwon-Do all over the world. Nowadays, it is possible to practice Taekwon-Do in almost every country in the world. The effort and dedication of Choi Hong Hi are the main reasons that the Koreans, who after World War II were in search of their own cultural background and national identity, are now greeted in every Dojang in the world when people bow to the Korean flag.

Basic principles of Taekwon-Do movements according to the founder
In his *Encyclopedia of Taekwon-Do* (1993), Choi Hong Hi described twelve basic principles, as listed below. These principles make Taekwon-Do a martial art, an aesthetic art, a science and a sport:

1. All movements have been designed to produce maximal strength in accordance with scientific formulas and the energy principle of motion theory.
2. The principles behind the techniques must be so clear that even those that have no knowledge of Taekwon-Do must be able to discern a correct movement from an incorrect movement.
3. The distance and angle of every movement must be exactly defined to achieve the greatest possible efficiency when it comes to attacks and defenses.
4. The goal and the method of every movement must be clear and simple to support the teaching- and learning process.
5. Rational teaching methods must be developed so that everyone – man and woman, young and old – may experience the advantages of Taekwon-Do.
6. The correct way of breathing must be determined in order to increase the speed of every movement and to avoid exhaustion.
7. It must be possible to attack every vital spot on the body, and it must be possible to defend against every variation of any attack.
8. Every instrument of attack must be defined and must be based on the composition of the human body.
9. Every movement must be easy to execute to give the student the opportunity to enjoy Taekwon-Do as a sport as well as a form of recreation.
10. Special attention must be paid to promoting good health and preventing injuries.
11. Every movement must be harmonious and rhythmic, so that Taekwon-Do is tasteful.
12. Every movement in the patterns must portray the personality and mental characteristics of the person after which the pattern was named.

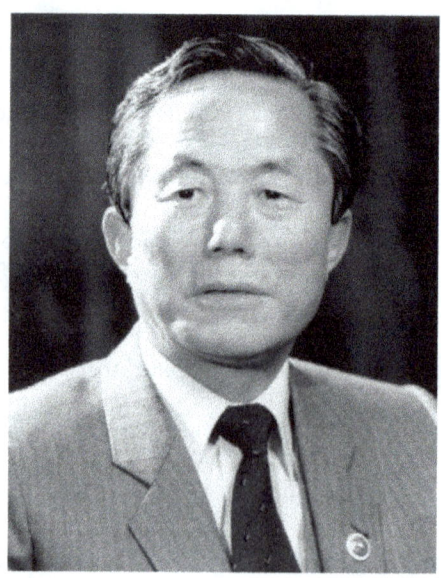

General Choi Hong Hi (1918-2002).

WTF and ITF

Towards the end of the 1960's General Choi was experiencing difficulties with factions within the South Korean Government, which eventually led to him seeking exile in Canada in 1972. His exile necessitated him giving up the presidency of the KTA but it was an action that ,would not only guarantee his own safety, but also that of Taekwon-Do. He established the headquarters of the ITF in Canada and during his time there continued to promote the original *Chang-Hun* Taekwon-Do internationally.

The newly-appointed regime in control of the KTA now decided to change its style, fighting techniques, style figures and rules. Style figures were now called *poomsae*, of which there were seventeen, and bore no resemblance to the patterns (*tuls*) that are found in *Chang-Hun* Taekwon-Do. Competition rules were amended so that armour could be worn, knockouts were allowed and you could forcefully hit each other during kicking techniques. The KTA did not allow hand techniques aimed at the head, which was contrary to the 'full contact' sparring of the ITF. In 1973, the KTA changed its name to the *World Taekwon-do Federation* (notice the lower-case 'd' in *do*) or WTF. This style of Taekwon-Do developed itself into a combat sport in direct conflict with the *martial art* that Choi Hong Hi had originally envisaged. This version of the sport became very popular, and in 1988 when the Olympics were held in South Korea, it was designated an Olympic sport (further increasing its popularity) which is why WTF Taekwon-do is now the style familiar to most people.

General Choi viewed his version of Taekwon-Do as a martial art for everyone, young or old, regardless of their race, beliefs or ideology. In 1980 General Choi travelled to Communist North Korea to promote Taekwon-Do as he dreamed that it perhaps could help to bring about the reunification of North And South Korea. South Korea, for their part, regarded these actions as a disgrace and throughout the 1980's promoted the idea that ITF Taekwon-Do was linked to communism, when in reality such political ideology has no place within the true meaning of Taekwon-Do.

The fundamental differences between the ITF and the WTF remain to this day. The ITF view Taekwon-Do as a martial art with its main focus on self-defense, whilst conquering your opponent from within yourself. The spiritual 'Do' in Taekwon-Do is of huge significance. The WTF, on the other hand, view it as a combat sport with the ultimate aim of defeating your opponent. These contrasting viewpoints show the clear difference between the two versions of Taekwon-Do.

The great irony in all of this is that the original ITF style of Taekwon-Do was developed by a South Korean General with assistance from South Korean soldiers within South Korea itself, who then went on to fight against communist North Korea during the civil war in the 1950's. Today North Koreans practice the original ITF style whilst South Koreans practice that of the WTF.

The shape of a turtle is shown in blue. In Southeast Asia, the turtle is sacred; symbolizing a long life.

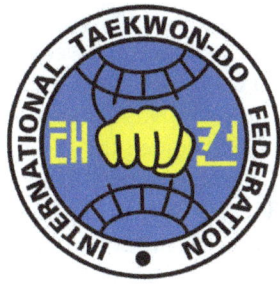

Figure 2.2 Emblem of the ITF

Up until his death in 2002, General Choi Hong Hi continued to spread the 'true' form of Taekwon-Do. This traditional style is known all over the world. After Choi Hong Hi's death, internal problems caused the ITF to split up into three organizations that all basically have the same manner of execution. ITF Royal Dutch is connected to the ITF of grandmaster Choi Jung Hwa (9th dan), son of the deceased founder.

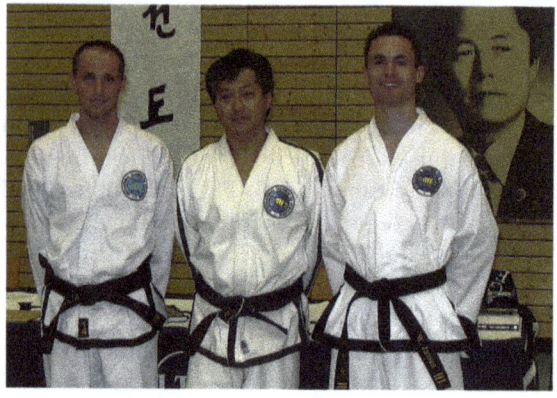

Grandmaster Choi Jung Hwa (center).

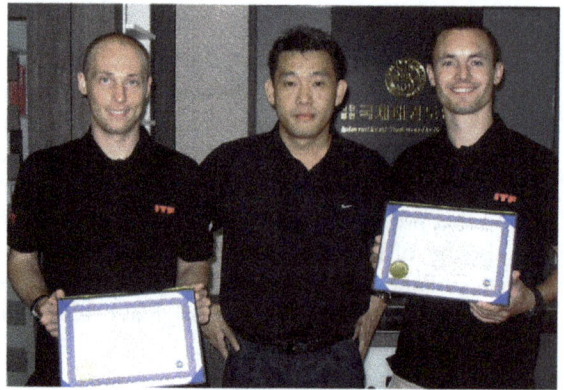

Secretary general ITF Korea, master Cj-Oh (center).

ITF Royal Dutch

In 1965, Kwon-Moo Gun (5th dan at the time) from Korea was the first one to teach Taekwon-Do in the Netherlands (in Venlo). In a sense, this was the way Taekwon-Do was introduced in the Netherlands. Six months later Kwon-Moo Gun was teaching in the cities of Oss, Nijmegen, and Enschede as well. Around the same time, Park Jong Soo (5th dan at the time) came to The Hague, the Netherlands. The two groups started cooperating and on May 29th, 1966, the Dutch Taekwon-Do Association (NTA) was founded. The NTA joined the ITF almost immediately. In 1968, founder General Choi Hong Hi, president of the ITF, paid his first visit to the Netherlands. The NTA has a rich history with many highs but some lows as well. It has proven to be impossible to have only one Taekwon-Do organization on a national level. In 1985, the NTA decided to part ways with the ITF and follow its own path. Among other things, this caused several schisms at the time. Contacts with grandmaster Choi Jung Hwa's ITF were not restored until the beginning of the 21st century, after the passing of the founder. Still, much remained unclear and there was a sense of unrest within the NTA concerning the direction it should take, which left the organization fruitless for decades.

At the end of 2009, the authors, together with Master Steve Zondag and Sabum Hennie Thijssen – who have been practicing Taekwon-Do since its early years in the Netherlands – have decided to take matters into their own hands. Their goal was to start a full-fledged traditional ITF Taekwon-Do organization with a clear active policy and international cooperation with mother organization ITF. On February 3rd, 2010, Master Steve Zondag, Sabum Hennie Thijssen, Sabum Paul van Beersum, and Sabum Willem Jansen signed the official opening document of ITF Royal Dutch in Bunnik.

Before the summer of 2010, ITF Royal Dutch has become the largest ITF grandmaster Choi Jung Hwa organization in the Benelux (Belgium, the Netherlands, and Luxemburg). ITF Royal Dutch has been acknowledged by the ITF world organization as the only INO (Independent National Organization)-certified organization of the ITF. This entails that ITF Royal Dutch is the mother organization and captain of ITF grandmaster Choi Jung Hwa Taekwon-Do in the Netherlands.

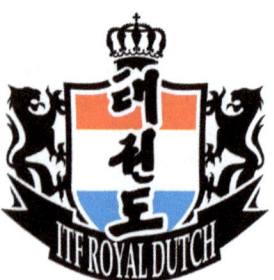

Figure 2.4 Emblem of the ITF Royal Dutch

ITF Royal Dutch is a foundation that mainly focuses on target groups that (want to) practice the form of Taekwon-Do as developed by the late General Choi Hong Hi, founder of Taekwon-Do. This is why ITF Royal Dutch associates itself with the ITF world organization of grandmaster Choi Jung Hwa, Choi Hong Hi's son. ITF Royal Dutch has a proactive policy that strives to maintain the techniques and philosophy of the ITF world organization.

One of the objectives of ITF Royal Dutch is to adequately and quickly dedicate itself to the diverse target groups that are directly or indirectly connected. Everyone that practices this inspiring art should be able to mentally and physically develop themselves, regardless of age and rank. For this reason, ITF Royal Dutch is involved in the development, execution, and evaluation of practice sessions, seminars, and education. Depending on the target group, focus is on the further development of one or more competences that ITF Taekwon-Do possesses (knowledge, skills, and attitude). Furthermore, ITF Royal Dutch thoroughly prepares people for taking their dan promotion tests, teaching, or competing in matches (up to a global level). This corresponds to another objective of the ITF Royal Dutch, which is to be an intermediary, a bridge between people, alliances, organizations, and schools, the goal being to promote the ITF in a respectful manner with mutual feelings of trust.

Working hard, providing appropriate information, trusting and respecting each other, and educating motivated instructors with characters that correspond to the tenets of Taekwon-Do will all be very significant in guaranteeing the continuity of the ITF Royal Dutch. This is also important to acquire challenging insights and to be able to ensure the guarantee of inspiring training sessions, seminars, and workshops in the field of ITF Taekwon-Do.

ITF Royal Dutch is comprised of a board and several committees:
- Competition Selection Committee;
- Referees Committee;

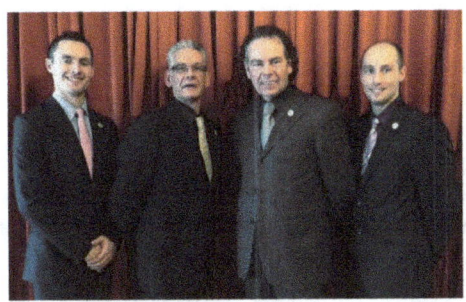

Founders and board members of ITF Royal Dutch.

- Teacher Training College Committee;
- Technical Education Committee;
- Dan Rank Committee.

Every committee consists of a number of certified experts in Taekwon-Do. Every committee has its own task. ITF Royal Dutch offers several national activities for its members, such as national and international championships and events, national technical instructions and instructions for competitions, teacher- and referee education, and national dan rank exams. ITF Royal Dutch also offers several activities for Taekwon-Do schools and students that are not associated with the foundation.

Taegeukgi

Taegeukgi is the name of the South Korean flag (see Figure 2.5), which has been mentioned before. The flag originates from 1882 and can be found in almost any Dojang where Korean martial arts (*Mudo*) are

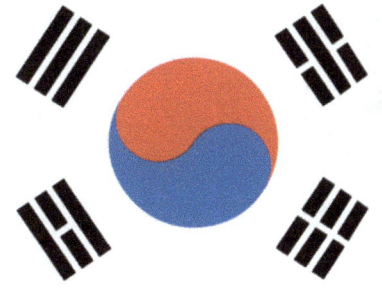

Figure 2.5 South Korean flag

practiced. This flag is highly symbolic for South Korea and its philosophy of life, which is represented in the martial arts. In that sense, the flag has become a symbol for Korean martial arts.

The fundamental color of the flag is white, which symbolizes 'peace'. In the corners of the flag there are four 'trigrams'; a combination of interrupted and uninterrupted lines. Originally, Chinese philosophy has eight trigrams or pillars. These represent the basic elements (fire, water, earth, wood, etc.). These elements in turn represent Taoist wisdoms, which mainly concern health, harmony, long life, and medical science. Also, the trigrams represent the opposite principles of light and dark ('eum' - 'yang'). The locations of the trigrams on the flag symbolize the four points on a compass. The trigram in the lower left corner symbolizes the sunrise in the east. The trigram in the upper left corner represents the sun at its highest point of the day in the south. The trigram in the upper right corner represents the sun as it moves westward. The trigram in the lower right corner symbolizes the total darkness, when the sun is in the north. Together, these trigrams represent the mysteries of the universe. For more information on the trigrams, the authors would like to refer you to the consulted and recommended literature in Appendix 3.

The four trigrams in the Korean flag represent:

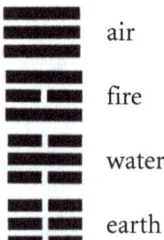

air

fire

water

earth

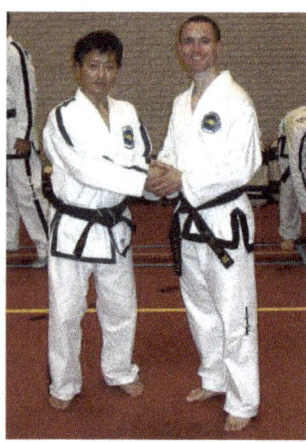

President ITF Grandmaster Choi and Willem Jansen.

In the middle there is a yin yang symbol (*eum-yang* in Korean) in blue (bottom) and red (top). In Korean, this circle is called *Taeguk*. This circle originates from Taoism and symbolizes the source of everything in the universe. Blue (*eum*) represents all negative forces and (feminine) principles. Red (*yang*) represents all positive forces and (masculine) principles. These forces, principles, or aspects, are based on cooperation and resistance. In eum, there is yang, and in yang, there is eum. Together they make up the Taoist vision on life and the universe. Therefore, the Taeguk symbolizes how one sees and understands himself and the world, in relation to the constant movement (or energy) within the universe. All of this comes together in the 'Do' in Taekwon-*Do*. Consequently, there is a distinct connection between the Korean flag, Oriental philosophy, and Taekwon-Do.

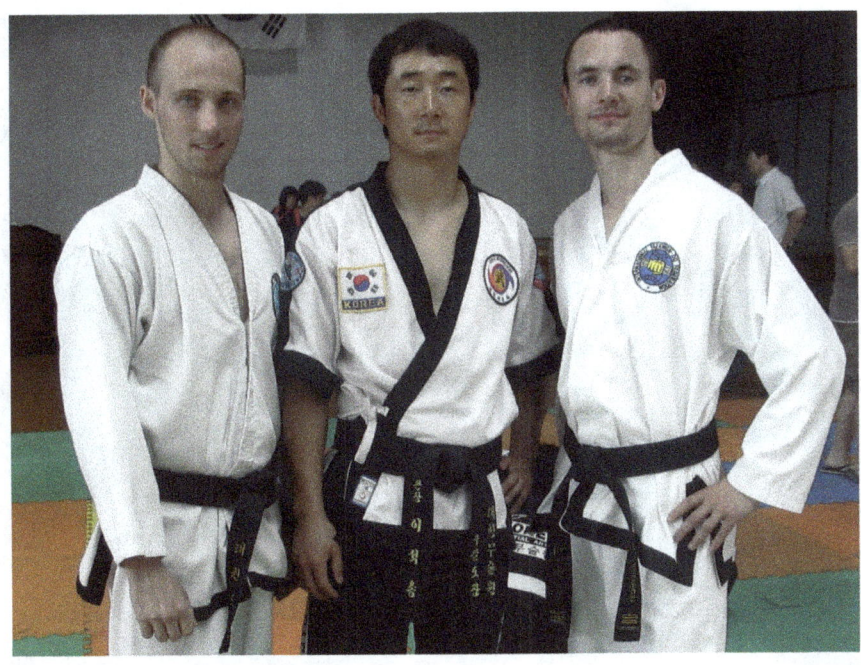

Paul van Beersum and Willem Jansen with the local Hapkido Master after their Taekwon-Do demonstration at a martial-arts festival South Korea.

Working out with Master Lee from Japan, Tokyo at a special instructors seminar.

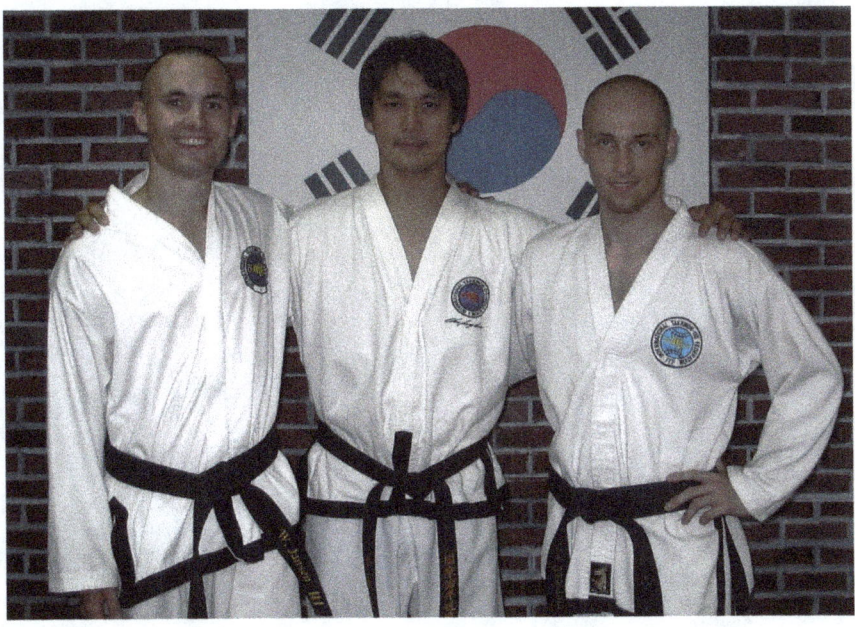

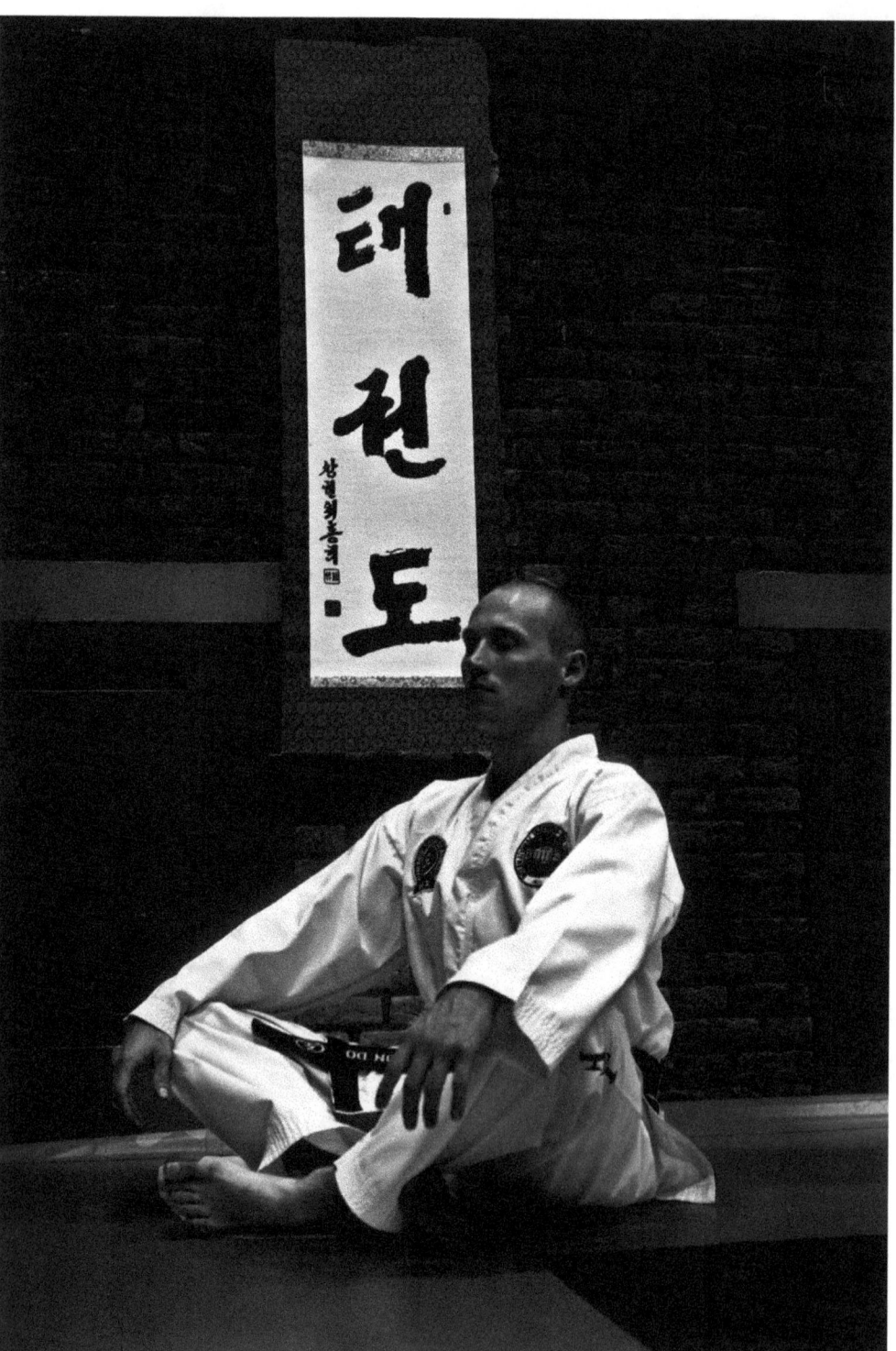

3. TAEKWON-DO, A WAY OF LIFE

3.1 A closer look at Taekwon-Do

Taekwon-Do is a Korean martial art that does not use weapons. The word 'Taekwon-Do' can be divided into three words:

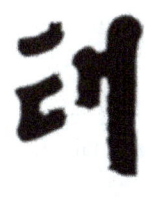

Tae
Literally translated, it means jumping or flying, kick or break with foot.

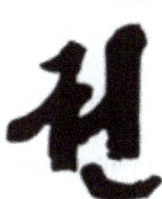

Kwon
Fist. Mainly for punching, or destroying with hand or fist

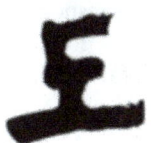

Do
Way or method.

Taekwon-Do is a Korean way of unarmed fighting and mental training. Arms and legs are used for blocking, avoiding, striking, punching, thrusting and kicking; quickly eliminating the opponent(s) is the goal. The Taekwon-Do techniques are based on modern physical science. Through intense mental and physical training, one can develop great powers with their body. This is why one who practices Taekwon-Do is able to break several stones with one strike or eliminate an opponent with one single technique.

However, Taekwon-Do is more than a way of fighting. This is because of the personal philosophy of the founder and the *Do* that is so clearly present in the traditional form of Taekwon-Do. It is hard to describe the word 'Do' sometimes, especially to the Western frame of mind. Do is more than just a method; it is a traditional East Asian way of life. It signifies existing with a good attitude in life or a good mental attitude. Therefore, it is very important *how* one walks the path, or the way. Practicing Taek-

> **FEATURES OF DO**
> FOCUSED ON:
> self-discipline
> physical perseverance
> spiritual, mental and personality development
> striving and searching for perfection of technique and exercise (zen)
> etiquette and respect
> self-development
> rest, meditation, and concentration
> increasing sense of self-worth and self-confidence
> lifelong activity
> art of life

won-Do makes it possible to develop the body, the soul, and the spirit, in harmony with nature. In that sense, Taekwon-Do is also a way of life. For example, think of Taekwon-Do as health exercises for the body and the mind, the pedagogical value of Taekwon-Do, or learning how to defend oneself. A serious student of Taekwon-Do occupies himself with this art every day. It is not just about training regularly, teaching, or studying the different techniques. On the surface, Taekwon-Do seems like a technical sport, but beneath that lies a lifestyle based on ethics and morals. It is about the way one perceives life and lives life. The beginning student is usually occupied with learning different self defense techniques, and the young dan rank holder is often occupied with matches. As mentioned before, Taekwon-Do and the way of life that accompanies it truly start after acquiring the black belt. The authors have seen how people are often involved with the element of sparring, and not with the traditional ways of practicing and the philosophies and tenets that are behind it.

What are the tenets and Asian philosophy of Taekwon-Do exactly? The founder of Taekwon-Do has included some tenets – or more simply put, objectives – in his *Encyclopedia* (in calligraphy in Figure 3.1). Furthermore, he has written a separate volume on Asian philosophy. The tenets of Taekwon-Do are listed below. Apart from physical training, every student will have to train themselves on a spiritual level.

Tenets

Ye Ui
This means courtesy or modesty. According to the founder, those who practice Taekwon-Do must put effort into practicing the aspects of courtesy that are written below, both in- and outside the Dojang, in order to develop a noble character.

1. Promoting the energy with mutual consent.
2. Being ashamed of one's own sins and despising other people's sins.
3. Being polite to each other.
4. Encouraging feelings of justice and humanity.
5. Distinguishing instructor from student, senior from junior, and elder from younger.
6. Behaving according to etiquette.
7. Respecting the possessions of others.
8. Handling business with reason and honesty.
9. Omitting to receive or give a questionable gift.

Yom Chi
This means integrity or honesty. A Taekwon-Do student must be able to distinguish right from wrong and, if necessary, to be ashamed. The founder gives several examples in which integrity is missing.

1. An instructor who presents themselves and the art incorrectly or shows incorrect techniques to their student because of a lack of knowledge or apathy.
2. A student who presents themselves incorrectly by preparing materials for breaking techniques during demonstrations.
3. An instructor who camouflages bad techniques with luxurious training facilities and false flattering of their students.
4. A student who asks or tries to obtain a dan rank from their instructor.
5. A student who acquires their rank or boosts their ego in order to feel powerful.
6. An instructor who teaches and promotes their art in order to pursue materialistic goals.
7. A student whose actions do not correspond with their words.
8. A student who is ashamed to ask for the opinion of their juniors.

In Nae
This means perseverance. Characteristics of a true Taekwon-Do student are persistence and inflexibility. Perseverance and determination are necessary to become a good Taekwon-Do student. It takes years of exercise to master a technique. In daily life, perseverance is very significant as well; life also has its obstacles and adversities. To overcome these difficulties, perseverance is often needed. Chinese philosopher Confucius stated: 'one who is impatient

in trivial matters can seldom achieve success in matters of great importance'.

Guk Gi

This means self-control. It is of great importance that a Taekwon-Do student has the discipline to control himself, since he has a wide range of techniques to injure someone. Self-control is significant not only in competitive or fighting circumstances, but also in daily life. Without self-control, one can cause unjust harm or end up in a dangerous or complicated situation. Therefore, self-control does not only apply to fighting techniques, but also to attitude. A Taekwon-Do student can be a source of peace. Chinese philosopher Lao Zi said the following about self-control: 'the term stronger is the person who wins over oneself rather than someone else.'

Baekjul Boolgool

This stands for the indomitable spirit or courage in life. A true Taekwon-Do student stands for his words and his principles. Adversities or injustice are combated without fear or doubt. Chinese philosopher Confucius has said: 'It is an act of cowardice to fail to speak out against injustice.'

These tenets are the ultimate goal of Taekwon-Do. Taekwon-Do is meant to develop oneself as a noble and pure person. Next, there is a manual, written by the founder in his personal philosophy. This serves as a basis for Taekwon-Do:

1. Be willing to go where the going may be tough and do the things that are worth doing even when they are difficult.
2. Be gentle to the weak and tough to the strong.
3. Be content with what you have in money and position but never in skills.
4. Always finish what you begin, be it big or small.
5. Be a willing teacher to anyone regardless of religion, race, or ideology.
6. Never yield to repression or threat in the pursuit of a noble cause.
7. Teach attitude and skill with action rather than words.

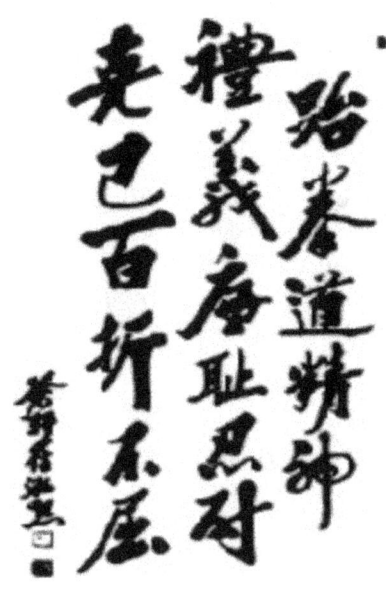

Figure 3.1 The tenets of Chang-Hun Taekwon-Do, as written by the founder in calligraphy.

8. Always be yourself even though your circumstances may change.
9. Be the eternal teacher who teaches with the body when young, with words when old, and by moral precept even after death.

Through serious training in physical as well as spiritual aspects of Taekwon-Do one develops oneself to a skilled martial artist.

3.2 The pedagogical value of Taekwon-Do

When staying in the course of the aforementioned tenets, the link to the pedagogical value of Taekwon-Do is easily established.

Opinions on the influence that martial arts have on behavior are greatly divided. The media have a great influence on these opinions, through news paper articles or action movies for example. Much scientific research has been done about the connection between aggression, defensibility, and combat sports. It is not surprising to hear that some traditional forms of martial arts bring about certain positive psychosocial changes. These positive changes are not as strongly present when it comes to modern (competitive) combat sports. Therefore, there is a great difference between combat *sports* and martial *arts*[2].

The way in which Taekwon-Do is being practiced causes a positive self-image, an increase in self-confidence, and a decrease in uncontrolled aggression. Aside from these effects, there are also positive physical effects in practicing Taekwon-Do. For example; an increase in speed, coordination, balance, equilibrium, stamina, force, and reactive power. In short, Taekwon-Do improves both physical and mental health. Positive psychosocial effects of Taekwon-Do are:

- **perseverance;**
- **loyalty;**
- **sincerity;**
- **self-control;**
- **decrease in fear;**
- **self-confidence;**
- **decrease in aggression;**
- **positive self-image;**
- **independence.**

These positive character traits are developed through traditional training methods and distinctive etiquette. Herein lies the foundation for the pedagogical value of Taekwon-Do. Traditional training methods focus on the training of fundamental basic exercises and the tuls. There is no specific emphasis on participation in competition. On the contrary; there is attention for meditation and the philosophy of Taekwon-Do. The main goal of Taekwon-Do is to positively influence the character (see Figure 3.2).

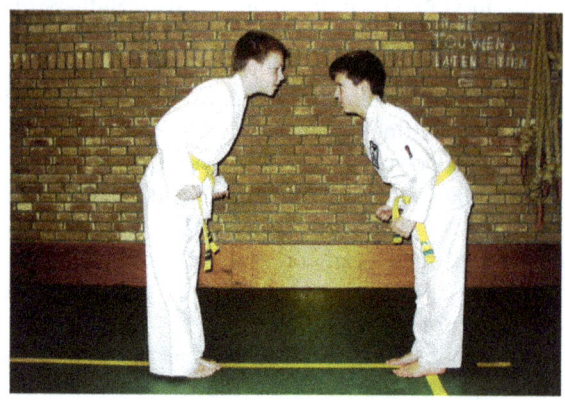

Figure 3.2 Positive influence on the character
Respect for each other, the instructor, the fellow man, and society.

In the previous paragraph the tenets of the founder have been discussed. In traditional Taekwon-Do it is not so much about learning to defeat the opponent as it is about learning to defeat the opponent in ourselves. The distinctive etiquette of Taekwon-Do is as significant as the training method.

There are no guarantees, since everyone is different. The instructor tries to keep this in mind as much as possible. Also, parents have their role as tutors. What is their parenting goal and how involved are they? How do parents deal with their child winning or losing a match, for example? What influence do friends have? What influence does society have? In short, the traditional goals of Taekwon-Do are clear, but the effect and results of the training are dependent on many factors. Taekwon-Do is made for life, so it would not be fair to the process to expect maximum results within only a few seasons.

---

2. Sources that are among those that the authors have consulted can be found in Appendix 3.

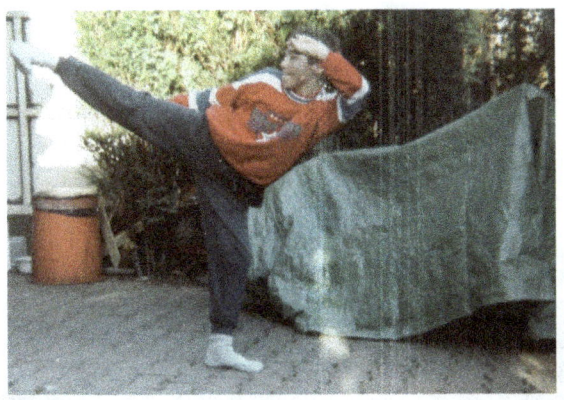 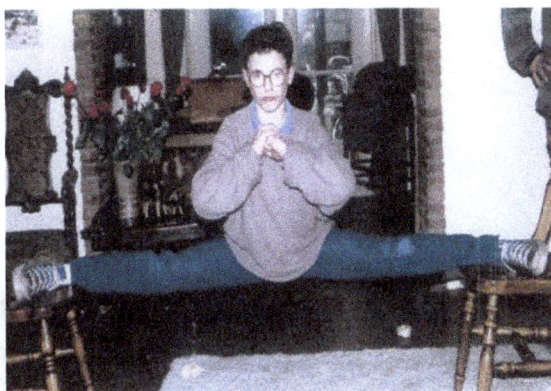

Van Beersum and Jansen at the age of 13.

The authors can confirm the aforementioned through their own experiences. The greatest compliment a Taekwon-Do teacher can receive is, for example, when parents tell them that their child is doing much better in school. However, this completely depends on the quality of the instructor and their vision. How do they conduct their lessons, and how is the bond between the instructor and the student? There is a difference between this relationship in the East and in the West. Think of hierarchy within Taekwon-Do. The teacher is a role model for respectful behavior. How does the teacher behave during a tournament? The teacher is responsible for the pedagogical climate. From this perspective, the authors feel that it is important that the Taekwon-Do organization, but also the teacher, takes responsibility for following an acknowledged Taekwon-Do teacher training program. It is the responsibility of the teacher to stay updated on the latest developments, to keep training, and to have an open mind but still be critical. Within ITF Royal Dutch there is the opportunity to take a course in three different levels (assistant teacher, teacher, head teacher). These courses are taught by 1st and 2nd degree teachers at an academic level. Parents should not be afraid to ask a Taekwon-Do organization if their instructors are qualified and if the organization is affiliated with a recognized Taekwon-Do association. Naturally, a parent wants to make sure their child is in good hands.

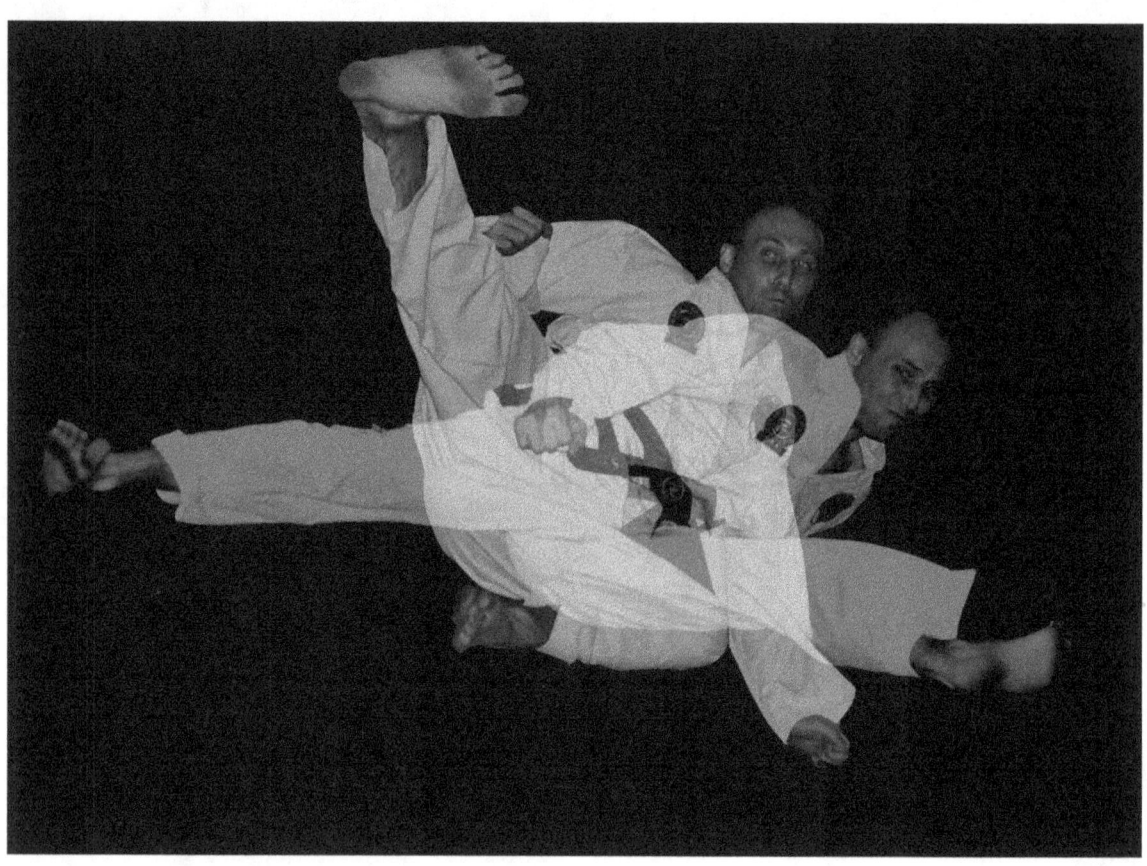

4. PHYSICAL ASPECTS OF TAEKWON-DO

In this chapter it is described which physical skills contribute to optimizing the practice of Taekwon-Do and practicing it to the fullest. Maintenance of the body and preparation for the practice of Taekwon-Do are important; aside from that the warming up, stretching, and the importance of good nutrition will be discussed.

4.1 Basic motor skills

While practicing Taekwon-Do, the body encounters several basic skills:

- strength;
- speed;
- endurance;
- flexibility.

Strength and endurance
During a match or fight, one who practices Taekwon-Do feels 'healthy tension': the body prepares itself for what is coming, the heart beats faster, and there is a sense of complete concentration. This alone requires energy, and there is not even movement yet. It is important that the body is in good condition; one good technique can end a fight. It is also possible that one is attacked or chased by several opponents at the same time. Strength and endurance are of great significance then. When these two skills are combined, strength endurance is created. Strength endurance determines how long a muscle or muscle group can persist a certain muscle exercise. Because of strength endurance one is able to muster up enough resistance when a fight lasts longer than expected.

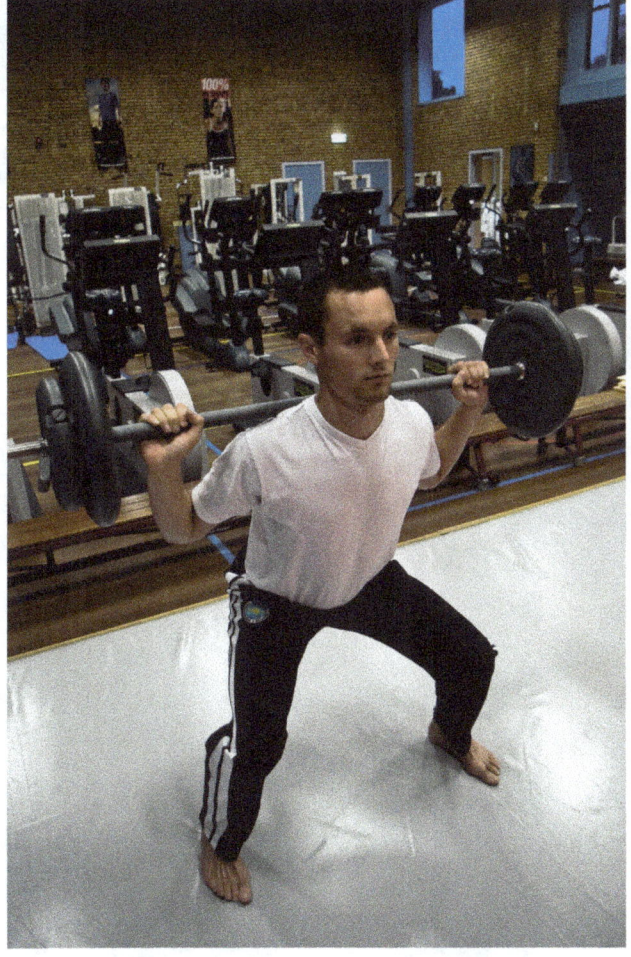

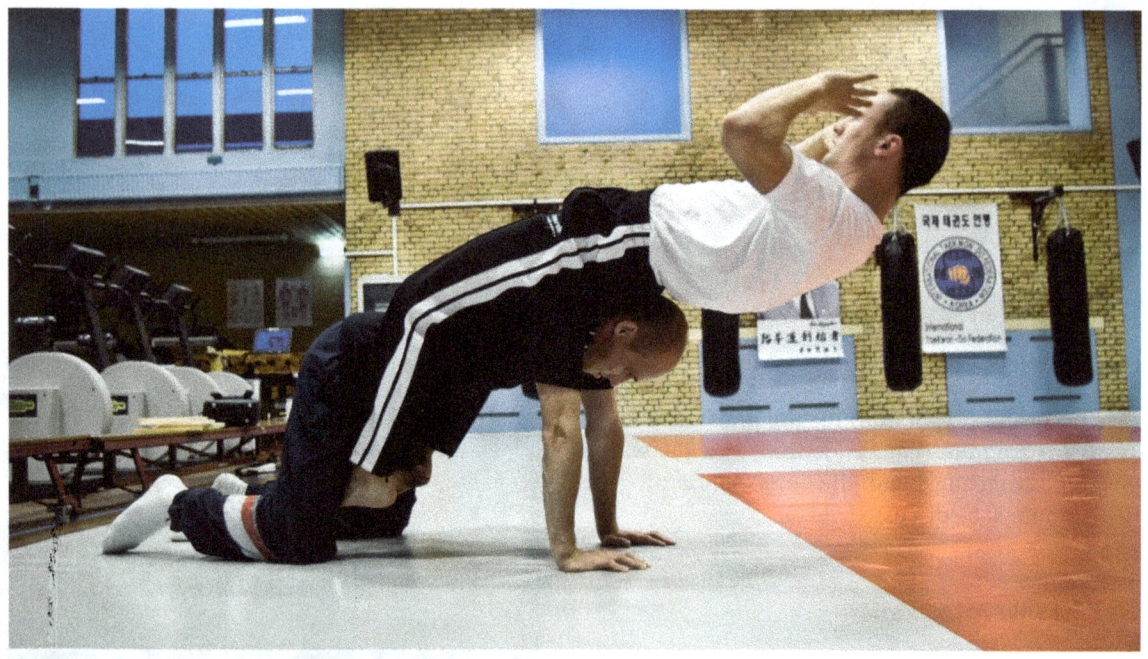

Speed

Speed can be very beneficial during a fight. One often thinks of the speed with which a technique is executed. However, there are different forms of speed:

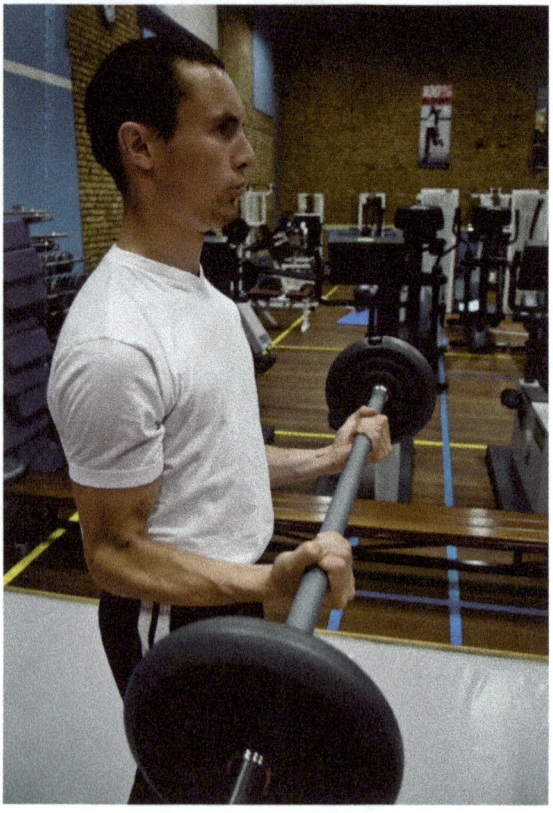

1. PERCEPTION SPEED: the speed with which one sees openings with the opponent, which one can respond to.
2. MENTAL SPEED: imentally choosing the correct movement as quickly as possible.
3. STARTING SPEED: taking initiative at the right moment, from the right position.
4. SPEED OF EXECUTION: the speed of moving, the chosen movement, and the effect of this.
5. ADAPTATION SPEED: the speed with which the direction of a movement can be changed. It is most important to maintain balance and relax.

There are several conditions that are needed to attain maximum speed:
- The body must be flexible and supple;
- The body must be in good shape;
- Physical and mental alertness;
- Imagination and foresight.

Flexibility

It has been mentioned before that it is important for the Taekwon-Do student that the body is flexible. Through regular stretching one will notice that certain techniques will be easier to execute, such as high kick techniques. It will become less difficult to perform a technique with precision. In paragraph 4.3 the attainment of the required flexibility will be discussed to a further extent.

The aforementioned motor skills can very well be trained. There are several different methods of training, such as endurance training, strength training, and interval training. Taekwon-Do is fast and explosive; a match or tul will not last longer than three minutes. It is possible though that several tuls or matches have to take place directly after one another. Adjust the training method to this; for example, practice many repetitions after each other. Strength endurance is reinforced by doing strength exercises (pushups, sit-ups) every 200 meters during running.

One should strive to become a little better with each training:
- jump even higher;
- punch even faster;
- kick even harder;
- become more flexible;
- do more repetitions;
- strive to be technically perfect.

When one does not have this dedication, the training can be considered wasted. It will take longer to achieve results and for the training to have any effect. It is possible to practice Taekwon-Do every day, although it is not sensible to put in maximum effort every day; rest and balance are important for the body as well. After an exhausting training on day one, training on day two could consist of stretching or the postponed execution of certain techniques. This is how the body prepares itself for the next intense training.

Aside from these training methods and basic skills, the technical training must not be forgotten. Remarks such as 'it's not working' or 'how do you do that?' are often heard. Oftentimes the answer is simply is: 'Training!' Make that same kick one hundred times, or repeat that tul over and over again. In short, invest time. A correct technical performance eventually saves energy and is good for the body. A prerequisite for this is good coordination, which is – among other aspects – a good cooperation between muscles, nerves, and senses. This way, the technique that is performed will have maximum force, speed, and precision. The key word is: repeat, repeat, repeat.

4.2 Warming up and cooling down

Before the actual training starts, it is important that the body is ready to train. The body is activated by warming up; the heart rate accelerates in order to provide enough oxygen and nutrition to the cardiovascular system, which enables the body to prepare itself for the training that will follow. In a specific warming up one can apply the movements that are also used during training. This is how the body is maximally prepared, both mentally and physically.

By cooling down, contrary to warming up, one makes the muscle tension and heart rate decrease gradually, so that the blood flow through the muscles is good and waste is drained from the body. This stimulates a fast recovery and diminishes the chance of aching muscles.

4.3 Stretching

Stretching has many advantages for the Taekwon-Doin. Everyone can learn how to stretch, regardless of age and flexibility. Most Taekwon-Do students stretch so that they become more flexible and are able to kick higher, in a more supple manner, and faster. The experienced Taekwon-Do student often stretches to bring mind and body together, and to achieve peace on the inside and the outside.

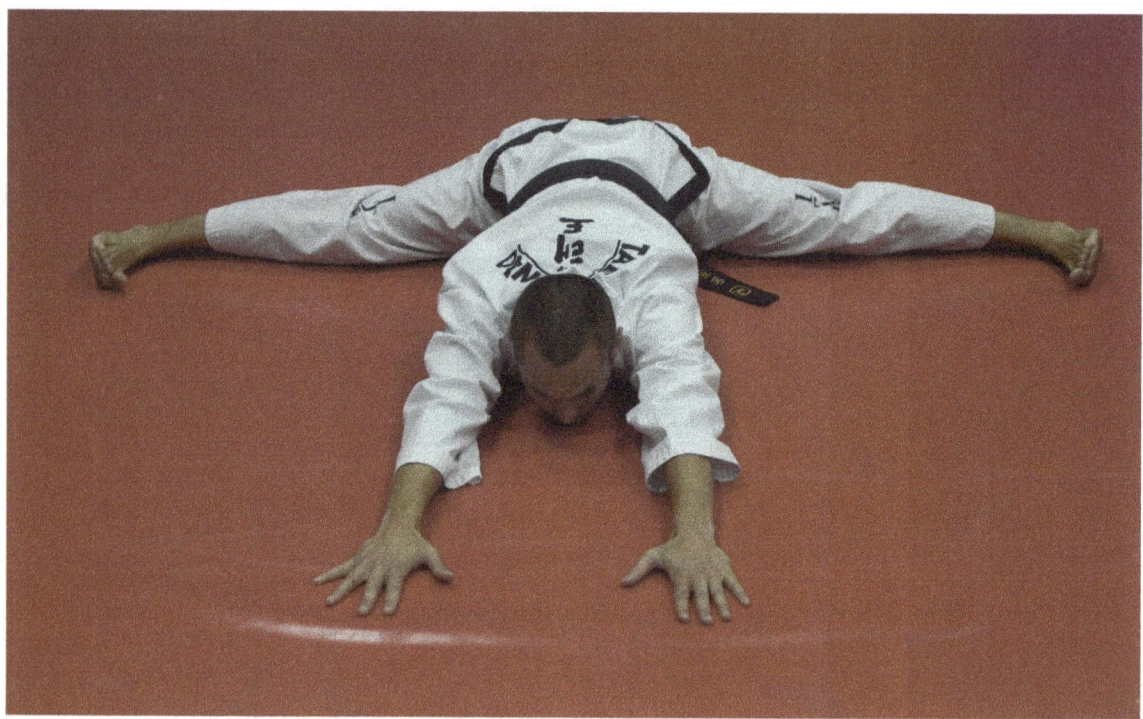

The authors recommend daily stretching. Consider it a simple daily exercise to increase flexibility in a relaxed fashion. A positive side effect is that it relaxes the mind after, for example, a hard day's work. Many forms of stretching originate from yoga. Several reasons for stretching are:

- Decrease of muscle tension;
- Relaxation of the body and peace of mind;
- Increase of flexibility and consequently an increase of movement possibilities;
- Prevention of injuries (resilience of a stretched muscle increases);
- Contribution to development of Chi;
- Increase in precision and control of Taekwon-Do techniques;
- Preparation, both mentally and physically, for the training;
- Improvement of blood circulation;
- Improvement of complete posture;
- Improvement of coordination;
- Last but not least: one gets to know themselves and set boundaries.

When should one stretch? It is important to at least stretch before and after a Taekwon-Do lesson. Stretching can be done anywhere and at any time. For example, one can stretch after waking up, while listening to music or watching television, during or after work, while waiting at a bus stop, etc. Apart from that, it does not mean that a good Taekwon-Do student is always stretching.

How should one stretch? There are different ways to stretch. Not every method is suitable for everyone. The safest method is the static stretch. The authors recommend this type of stretching to the beginning Taekwon-Do student. Next, several methods will be discussed briefly.

4. Physical aspects of Taekwon-Do   43

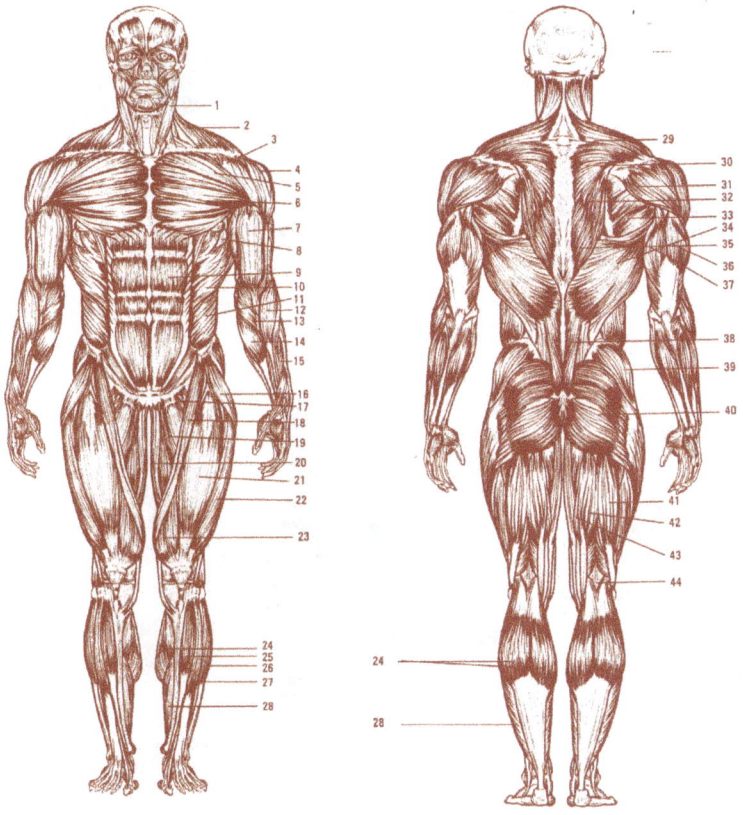

MUSCLES
1. Sternocleidomastoideus
2. Trapezius (upper)
3. Anterior deltoideus
4. Medial deltoideus
5. Clavicula pectoralis major
6. Sternus pectoralis major
7. Biceps brachii
8. Serratus anterior
9. Rectus abdominis
10. Underlying oblique
11. External oblique
12. Brachioradialis
13. Palmaris longus
14. Flexors
15. Extensors
16. Tensor fasciae latae
17. Pectineus
18. Sartorius
19. Adductor longus
20. Gracilis
21. Rectus femoris
22. Vastus lateralis
23. Vastus medialis
24. Gastrocnemius
25. Tibialis anterior
26. Peroneus longus
27. Extensors
28. Soleus
29. Levator scapulae (underlying)
30. Rhomboideus (underlying)
31. Posterior deltoideus
32. Trapezius (middle)
33. Teres major
34. Latissimus dorsi
35. Trapezius (bottom)
36. Triceps brachii (lateral)
37. Triceps brachii (long)
38. Erector spinae
39. Gluteus medius
40. Gluteus maximus
41. Biceps femoris
42. Semitendinosus
43. Semimenbranosus
44. Popliteus

Static method
With this method, the muscles are stretched without being forced. This is done by a light stretch which is held for 10 to 30 seconds. Relax after the light stretch and proceed with an increasing stretch. It is the same exercise, but a few centimeters further, until tension is felt again. Hold this tension for 30 seconds or longer. Perform these exercises calmly and controlled.

Next, several stretching exercises are shown. The layout is made based on the muscle groups on which the stretch focuses, although other muscle groups are also often stretched simultaneously.

Feet and ankle stretches

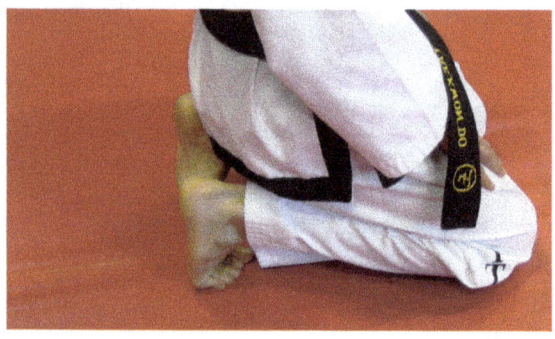

Figure 4.1 Ligaments and joints of the toes in particular.

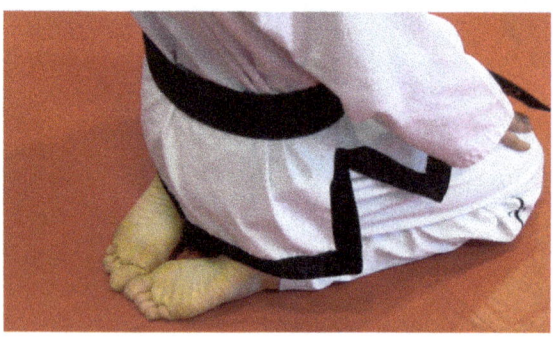

Figure 4.2 Ligaments and joints.

Front and back leg stretches

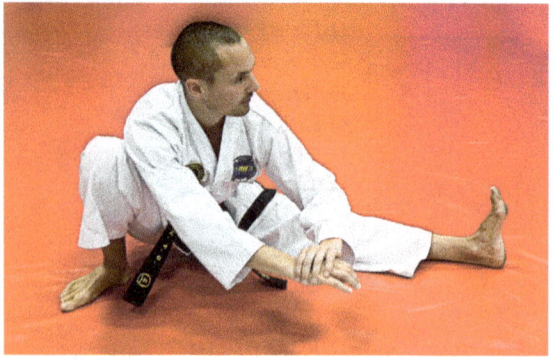

Figure 4.3 Hamstring = *m. (musculus) semimembranosus*, the *m. semitendinosus*, and the *m. biceps femoris*.

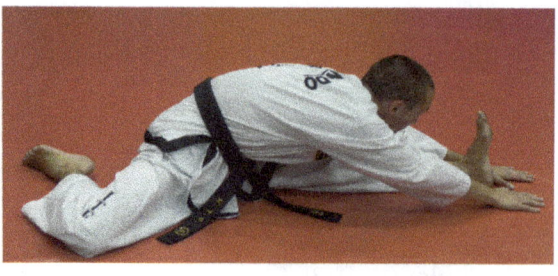

Figure 4.4 Hamstring = *m. semimembranosus*, the *m. semitendinosus*, and the *m. biceps femoris*.

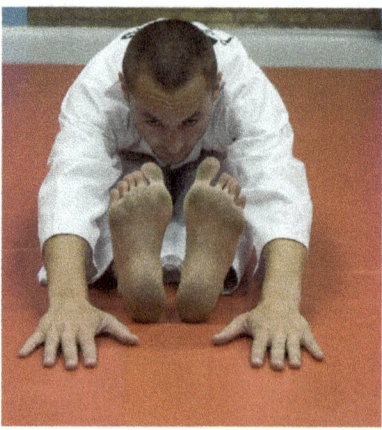

Figure 4.5 Hamstring = *m. semimembranosus*, the *m. semitendinosus*, and the *m. biceps femoris*. Iliocostalis muscle = *m. iliocostalis*.

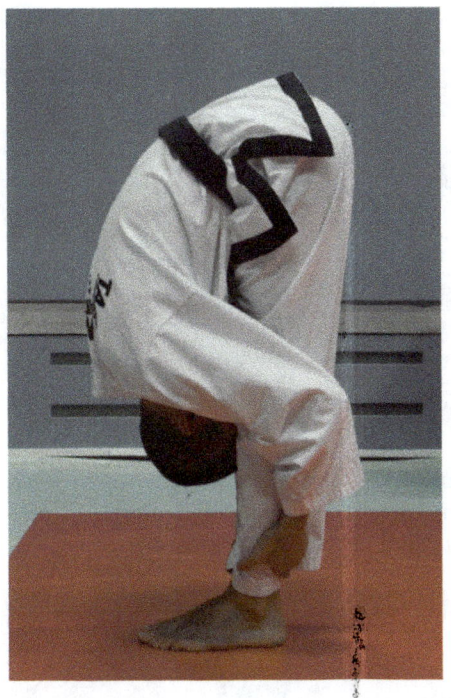

Figure 4.6 Hamstring = *m. semimembranosus, m. semitendinosus,* and *m. biceps femoris.*
Iliocostalis muscle = *m. iliocostalis.*

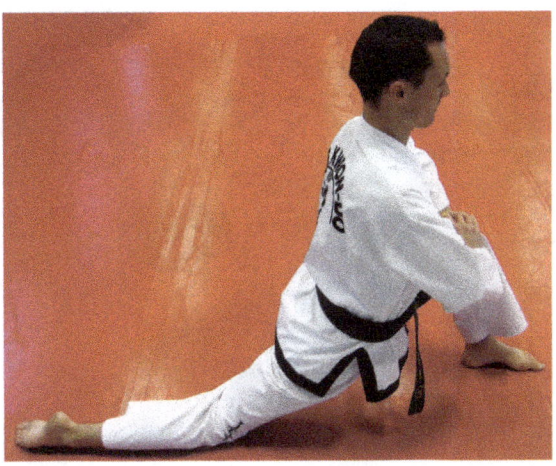

Figure 4.8 Dorsal hip muscles = *m. iliopsoas.*

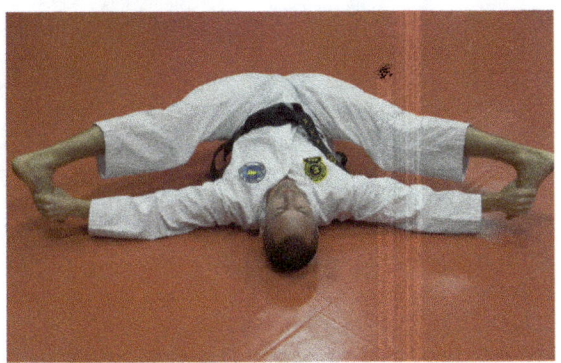

Figure 4.7 Hamstring = *m. semimembranosus,* the *m. semitendinosus* and the *m. biceps femoris.*
Iliocostalis muscle = *m. iliocostalis.*
Soleus muscle = *m. soleus.* Gastrocnemius muscle = *m. gastrocnemius.*

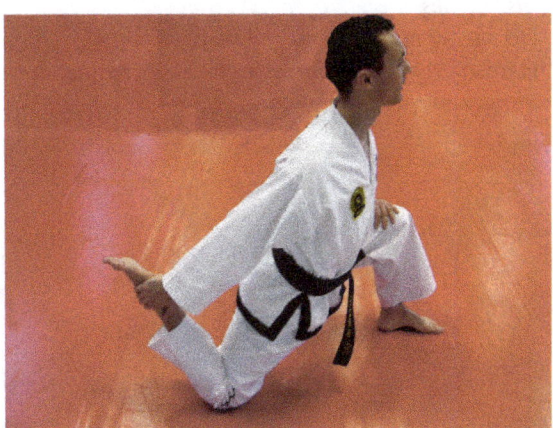

Figure 4.9 Quadriceps muscles = *m. rectus femoris, m.vastus medialis, m.vastus intermedius,* and *m. vastus lateralis.*
Dorsal hip muscles = *m. iliopsoas.*

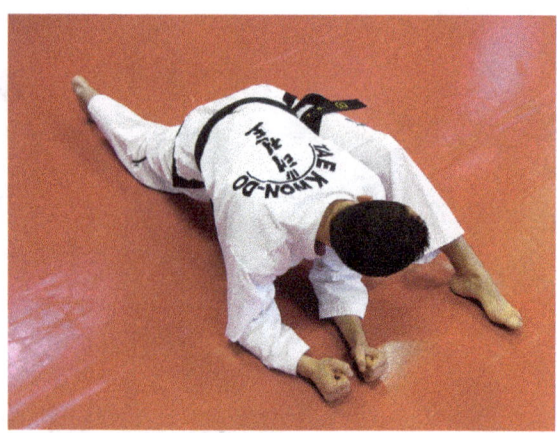

Figure 4.10 Quadriceps muscles = *m. rectus femoris, m.vastus medialis, m.vastus intermedius,* and *m. vastus lateralis.*
Dorsal hip muscles = *m. iliopsoas.*
Hamstring = *m. semimembranosus, m. semitendinosus,* and *m. biceps femoris.*

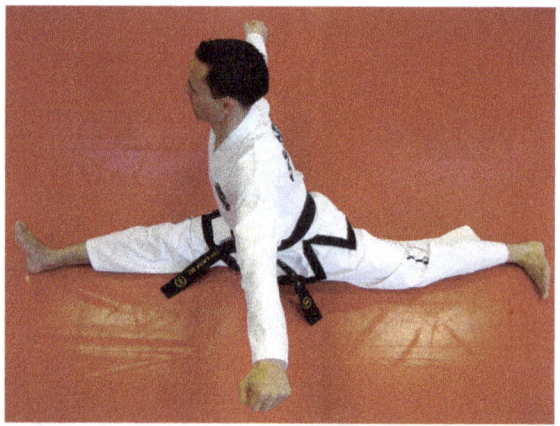

Figure 4.12 Dorsal hip muscles = *m. iliopsoas.*
Hamstring = *m. semimembranosus, m. semitendinosus,* and *m. biceps femoris.*

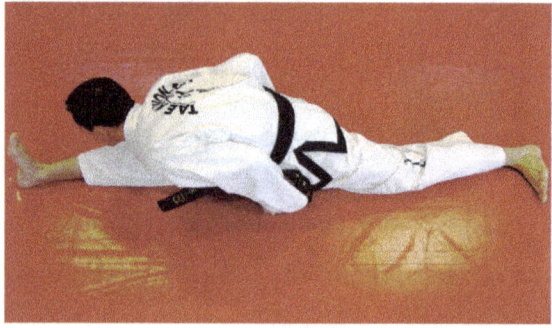

Figure 4.11 Dorsal hip muscles = *m. iliopsoas.*
Hamstring = *m. semimembranosus, m. semitendinosus,* and *m. biceps femoris.*

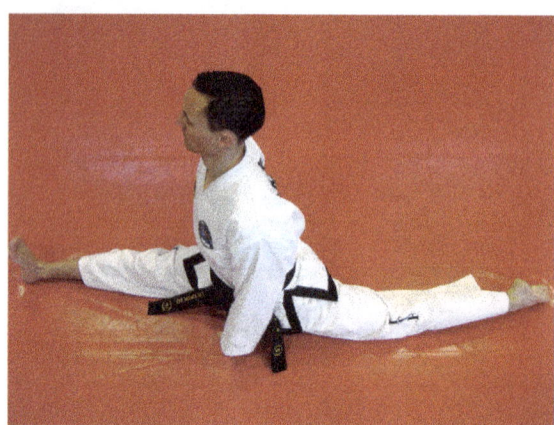

Figure 4.13 Quadriceps muscles = *m. rectus femoris, m.vastus medialis, m.vastus intermedius,* and *m. vastus lateralis.*
Dorsal hip muscles = *m. iliopsoas.*
Hamstring = *m. semimembranosus, m. semitendinosus,* and *m. biceps femoris.*

4. Physical aspects of Taekwon-Do 47

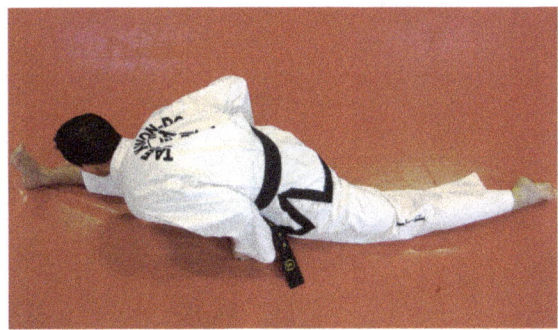

Figure 4.14 Quadriceps muscles = *m. rectus femoris, m.vastus medialis, m.vastus intermedius,* and *m. vastus lateralis.*
Dorsal hip muscles = *m. iliopsoas.*
Hamstring = *m. semimembranosus, m. semitendinosus,* and *m. biceps femoris.*

Inner thigh stretches

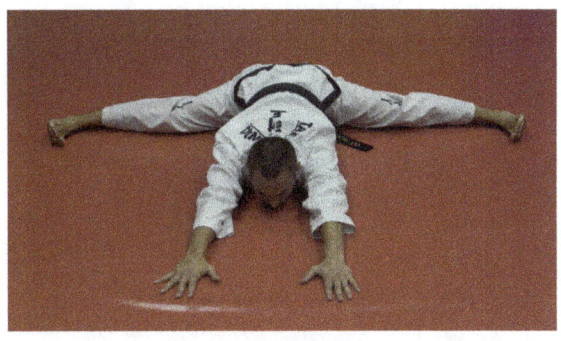

Figure 4.15 Adductors = *m. adductor magnus, longus* and *brevi, m. sartorius,* and *m. gracilis.*
Sartorius muscle = *m. sartorius.*

Lower back, hip joint and pelvic floor stretches

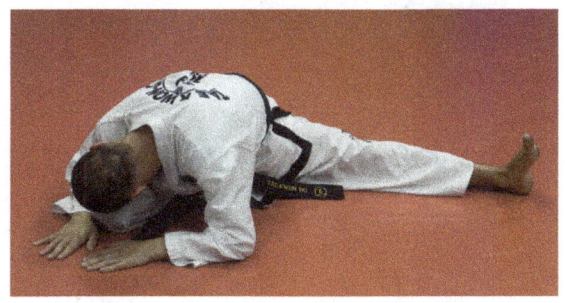

Figure 4.16 Erector spinae muscle = *m. erector spinae.*
Iliocostalis muscle = *m. iliocostalis.*
Gluteus maximus muscle = *m. gluteus maximus.*

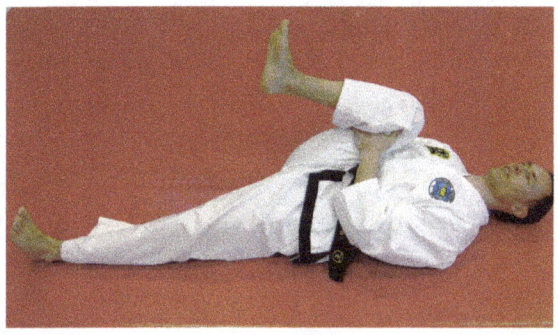

Figure 4.17 Gluteus maximus muscle = *m. gluteus maximus.*
Iliocostalis muscle = *m. iliocostalis.*
Hamstring = *m. semimembranosus, m. semitendinosus,* and *m. biceps femoris.*

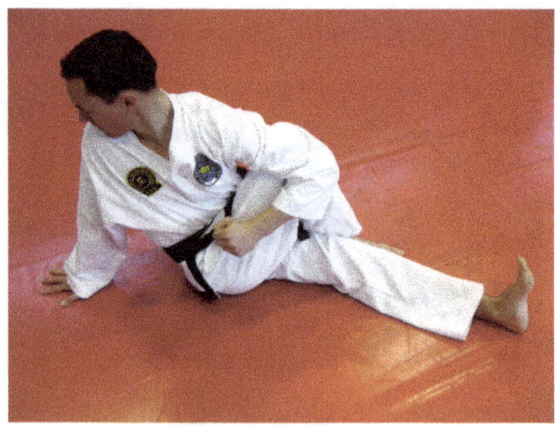

Figure 4.18 Gluteus maximus muscle = *m. gluteus maximus*.
Gluteus minius muscle = *m. gluteus minimus*.
Gluteus medius muscle = *m. gluteus medius*.
Tensor fascia lata (TFL) = *m. tensor fasciae latae*.

Back stretches

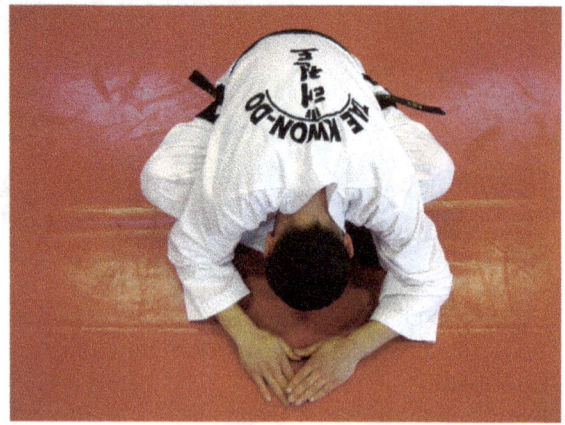

Figure 4.20 Broadest back muscle = *m. latissimus dorsi*.
Erector spinae muscle = *m. erector spinae*.
Iliocostalis muscle = *m. iliocostalis*.

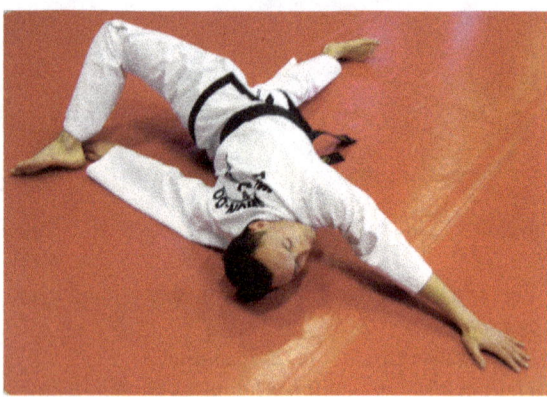

Figure 4.19 Broadest back muscle = *m. latissimus dorsi*.
Erector spinae muscle = *m. erector spinae*.
Ligaments and joints of the spinal column.

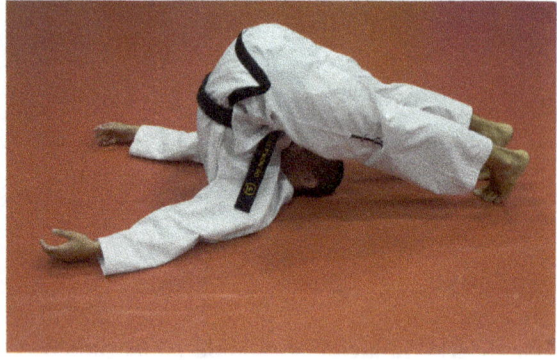

Figure 4.21 Broadest back muscle = *m. latissimus dorsi*.
Erector spinae muscle = *m. erector spinae*.
Iliocostalis muscle = *m. iliocostalis*.

Stomach and chest stretches

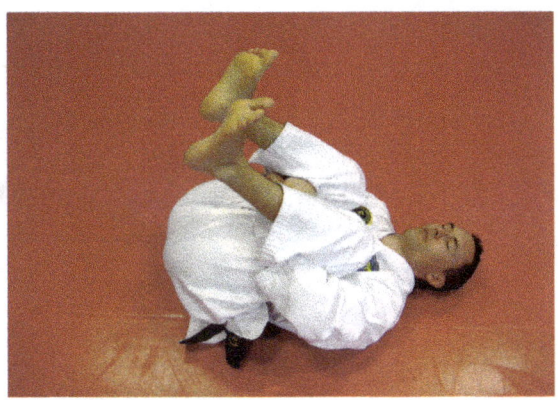

Figure 4.22 Broadest back muscle = *m. latissimus dorsi*.
Erector spinae muscle = *m. erector spinae*.
Iliocostalis muscle = *m. iliocostalis*.

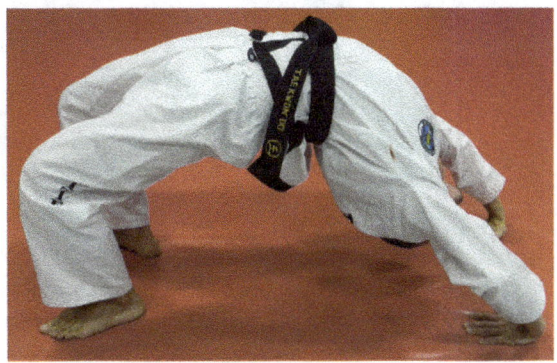

Figure 4.24 Rectus abdominus muscle = *m. rectus abdominis*. Abdominal internal oblique muscle = *m. obliquus internus abdominis*.

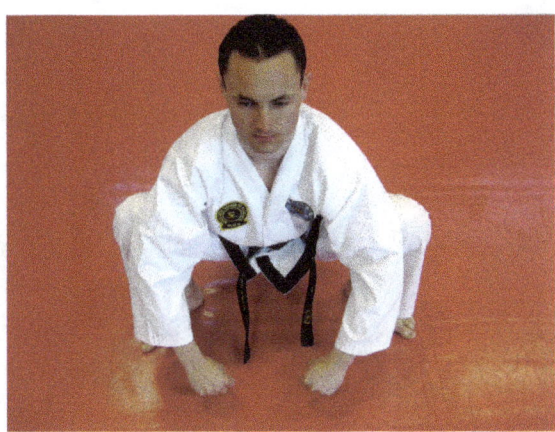

Figure 4.23 Broadest back muscle = *m. latissimus dorsi*.
Erector spinae muscle = *m. erector spinae*.
Iliocostalis muscle = *m. iliocostalis*.

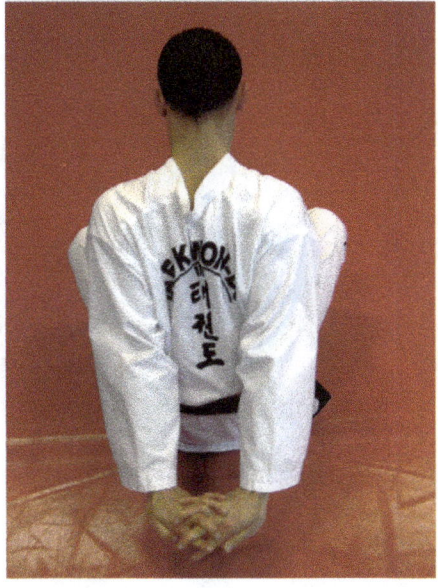

Figure 4.25 Pectoralis major muscle = *m. pectoralis major*. Deltoid muscle = *m. deltoideus*. Biceps = *m. biceps brachii*.

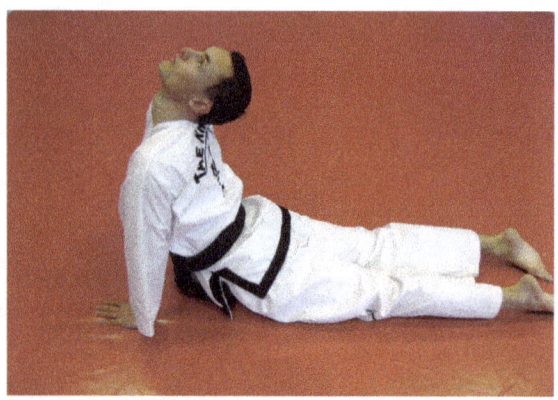

Figure 4.26 Rectus abdominus muscle = *m. rectus abdominis*.
Dorsal hip muscles = *m. iliopsoas*.

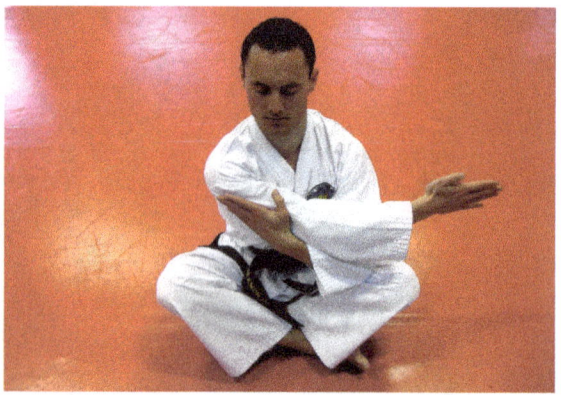

Figure 4.28 Deltoid muscle = *m. deltoideus*. Teres major muscle = *m. teres major*. Teres minor muscle = *m. teres minor*. Infraspinatus muscle = *m. infraspinatus*. Subscapularis muscle = *m. subscapularis*.

Arm, elbow, and shoulder girdle stretches

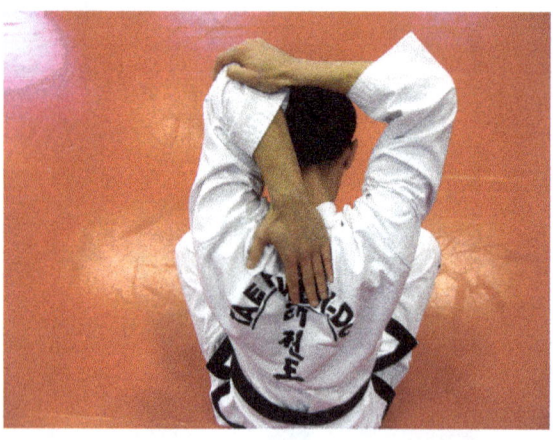

Figure 4.27 Triceps = *m. triceps brachii*.

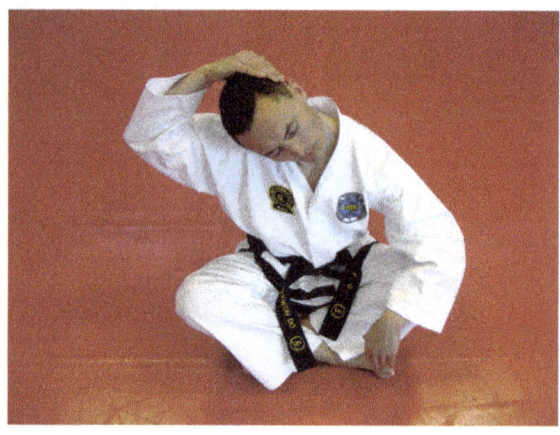

Figure 4.29 Rhomboid major muscle = *m. rhomboideus*.
Trapezius muscle = *m. trapezius*.

4. Physical aspects of Taekwon-Do

Ballistic method

The ballistic method, also dynamic or bouncing stretching, is a more forced type of stretching. The muscle is shortly put in the right position, but the stretch is not persisted. An increase in flexibility is possible via this method as well. However, the ballistic method takes up more energy and there is a greater chance of injuries (tissue damaging) and aching muscles, which is why the authors recommend static stretching for the beginning student.

Front and back leg stretches

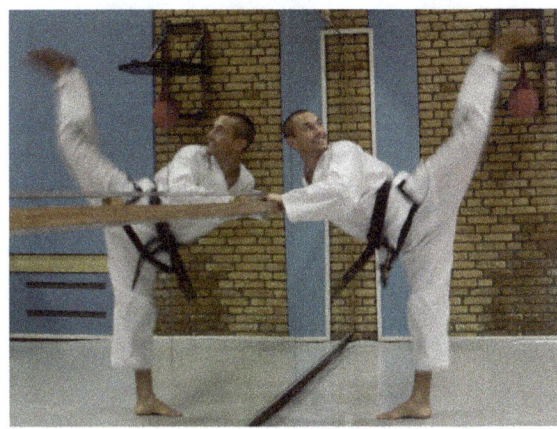

Figure 4.30 Dorsal hip muscles = *m. iliopsoas*.
Hamstring = *m. semimembranosus, m. semitendinosus*, and *m. biceps femoris*.
Quadriceps muscles = *m. rectus femoris, m.vastus medialis, m.vastus intermedius*, and *m. vastus lateralis*.

(Isometric) partner exercises

With the help of a partner, exterior force can be put on the muscles in a controlled manner. This is how, passively, a greater motion can be reached than one can actively achieve themselves. These exercises can be both static (isometric) and ballistic. A good collaboration with the partner and faith in the partner are required.

Front and back leg stretches

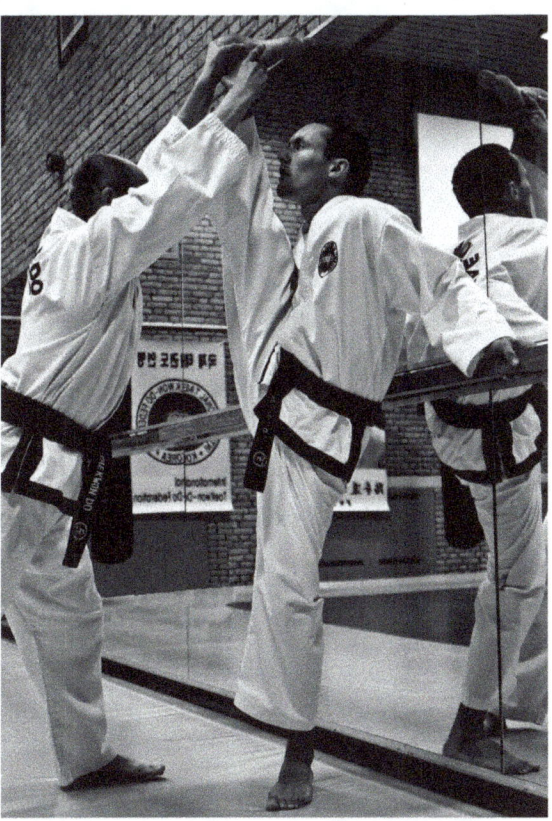

Figure 4.31 Hamstring = *m. semimembranosus, m. semitendinosus*, and *m. biceps femoris*.
Gluteus maximus muscle = *m. gluteus maximus*.

Inner thigh stretches

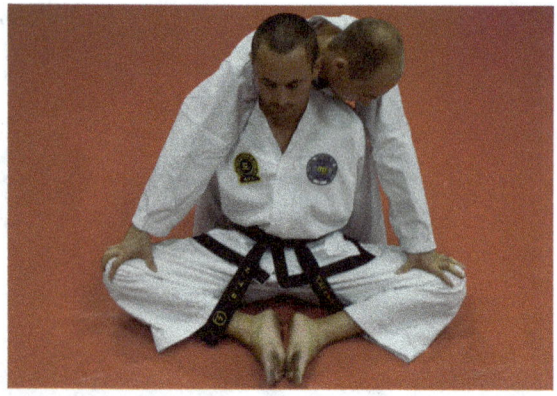

INTRODUCTORY LEVEL
Figure 4.32 Adductors = *m. adductor magnus*, *longus* and *brevi*, *m. sartorius*, and *m. gracilis*.

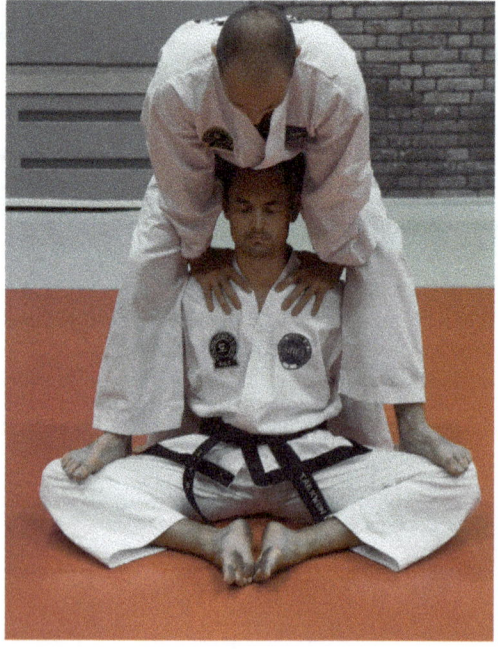

ADVANCED LEVEL
Figure 4.33 Adductors = *m. adductor magnus*, *longus* and *brevi*, *m. sartorius*, and *m. gracilis*.

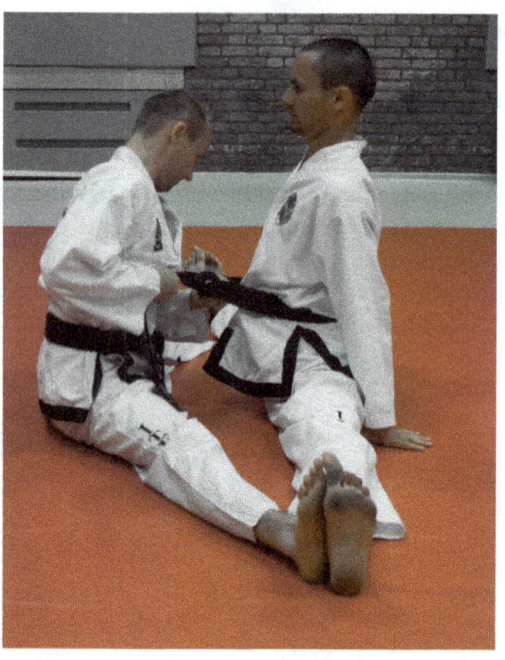

ADVANCED LEVEL
Figure 4.34 Adductors = *m. adductor magnus*, *longus* and *brevi*, *m. sartorius*, and *m. gracilis*.

Breathing and counting

This is very important while stretching. Ideally, breathing should be slow and rhythmic in order to reach complete relaxation. Preferably, exhaling takes place while bowing or slanting, whereas inhaling should take place while returning to a neutral stance. Do not hold your breath while stretching. When first starting out, it can be helpful to silently count while stretching, to make sure that the stretches are long enough.

As mentioned before, there are many opportunities to stretch. With a correct schedule of static exercises, that are performed for half an hour at least twice a week, an increase in flexibility can generally be noticed within five weeks. During the course of the training period, the duration of the stretches can be extended from 30 seconds to one minute, for example.

4.4 Nutrition

Make sure there is balance, not only in the frequency of training, but also in your nutrition. Whatever you burn while training must be replenished. Make sure that the body receives enough, and especially the right kind of nutrition when intense training takes place.

On average, a male needs 3000 calories a day and a woman needs 2400 calories. It is important to have a good balance of carbohydrates, fats, proteins, and vitamins. These are found in potatoes, rice, meat, dairy, and fruit. It is best to have a maximum of three main meals. Do not skip breakfast, and eat something small in between meals three or four times a day.

A *calorie* is the amount of energy that is needed to warm up one gram of pure water by 1 degree Celsius, at a pressure of a standard atmosphere. 1000 calories is 1 kilocalorie (kcal). Basically, (kilo)calories are the energy, the fuel, that the body needs to function. This energy is also defined in joules. 1 kilocalorie = 4184 joules, or 4.184 kilojoules (kJ).

Five rules of nutrition

1. EAT A VARIED DIET
There is not one particular food that contains all essential nutrients. Eating varied is necessary to obtain all essential nutrients. Moreover, the risk of ingesting any unhealthy elements is spread.

2. EXERCISE AND DO NOT EAT TOO MUCH
To maintain a healthy weight, is it significant to eat healthy and varied foods that do not contain too many calories, and to exercise regularly. A healthy bodyweight reduces the risk of chronic diseases. An overweight person has a higher risk of cardiovascular diseases, diabetes, and certain types of cancer. Not eating too much also means watching one's salt intake and alcohol intake.

3. LESS SATURATED FAT
Limiting the intake of saturated fat reduces the risk of cardiovascular diseases. However, fat is necessary as a source of unsaturated fatty acids, vitamins A, D, and E, and energy. Therefore, one should choose foods that contain unsaturated fat. Eating fish twice a week (with fatty fish at least once a week) is significant because of the healthy fatty acids that fish contains.

4. LOTS OF FRUIT, VEGETABLES, AND BREAD
Healthy nutrition contains great portions of vegetables, fruit, and bread. These foods are high in fiber and, taking into account their mass and weight, provide few calories and much nutrients. Therefore, one cannot easily eat too much. This is important for those watching their weight. Also, a high intake of fruit and vegetables reduces the risk of chronic diseases.

5. SAFETY
Foods can contain unhealthy elements and bacteria. Our food has never been this safe, but food that is 100% safe does not exist. At home, consumers are responsible for the safety of their food. By taking some simple measures, infections and diseases – the risk of food poisoning for example – can be reduced or prevented.

Important product groups are:

1. Fruit and vegetables
Important because of: vitamins, such as vitamin C and folic acid, minerals such as potassium, fibers, and bioactive elements.

2. Bread, grains, potatoes, rice, pasta, and legumes
Important because of: carbohydrates, proteins, B vitamins and minerals such as iron.

3. Dairy, meat, fish, eggs, and meat substitutes
Important because of: proteins, minerals such as iron and calcium, B vitamins, and fatty acids from fish.

4. Fats and oil
Important because of: vitamins A, D, and E, and essential fatty acids.

5. Drinks
Important because of: water.

It is not the purpose of this book to give dietary advice, nor to be exhaustive in providing nutritional rules. By offering this information, the authors hope to provide an insight in composing a healthy, balanced diet.

The energy that a resting body requires is acquired from carbohydrates and fat. During heavy and explosive exercise, mainly carbohydrates are burned by the body (which does not mean that there is no fat burning at all). This supply of carbohydrates usually 'wears out' after 60 to 90 minutes. This is why food that is rich in carbohydrates can have a positive effect on one's performance. It can be useful to replenish this source after a workout. This way, the body can heal quicker and easier before the next workout. Carbohydrates can also be taken before a workout, but this should be done several hours in advance, to prevent having to start exercising on a full stomach.

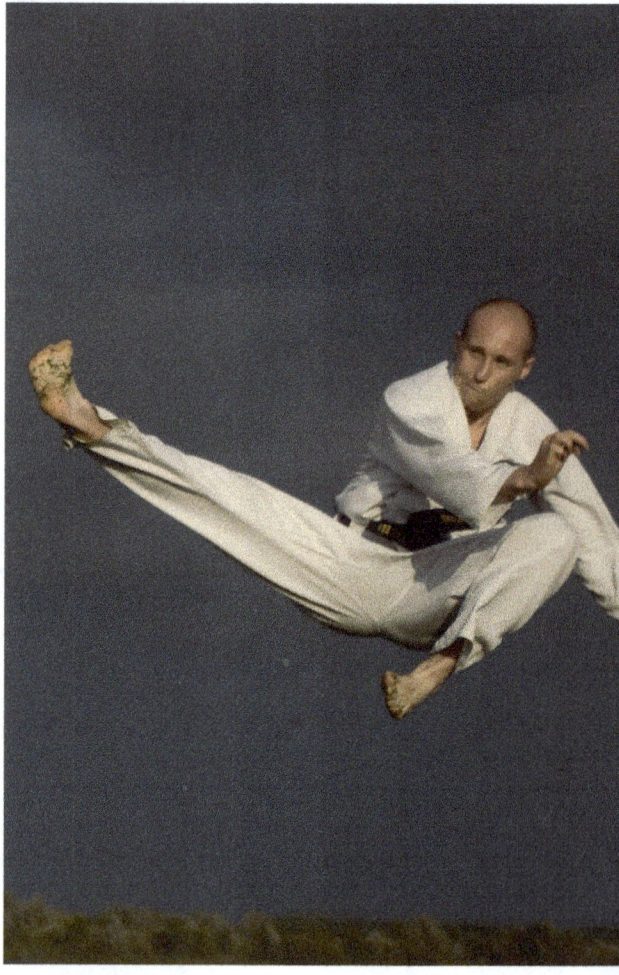

Twimyo Bituro Chagi.

4. Physical aspects of Taekwon-Do

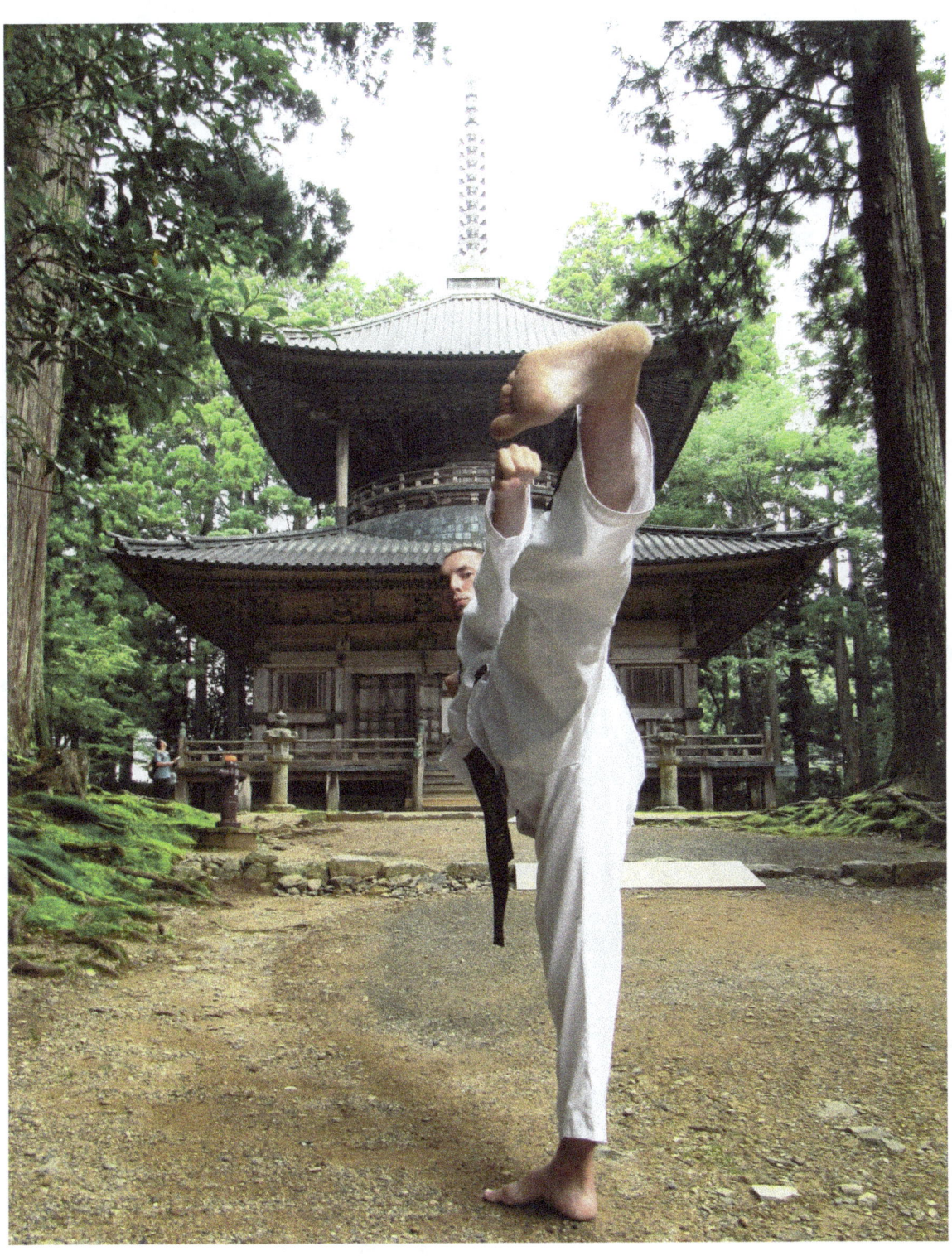

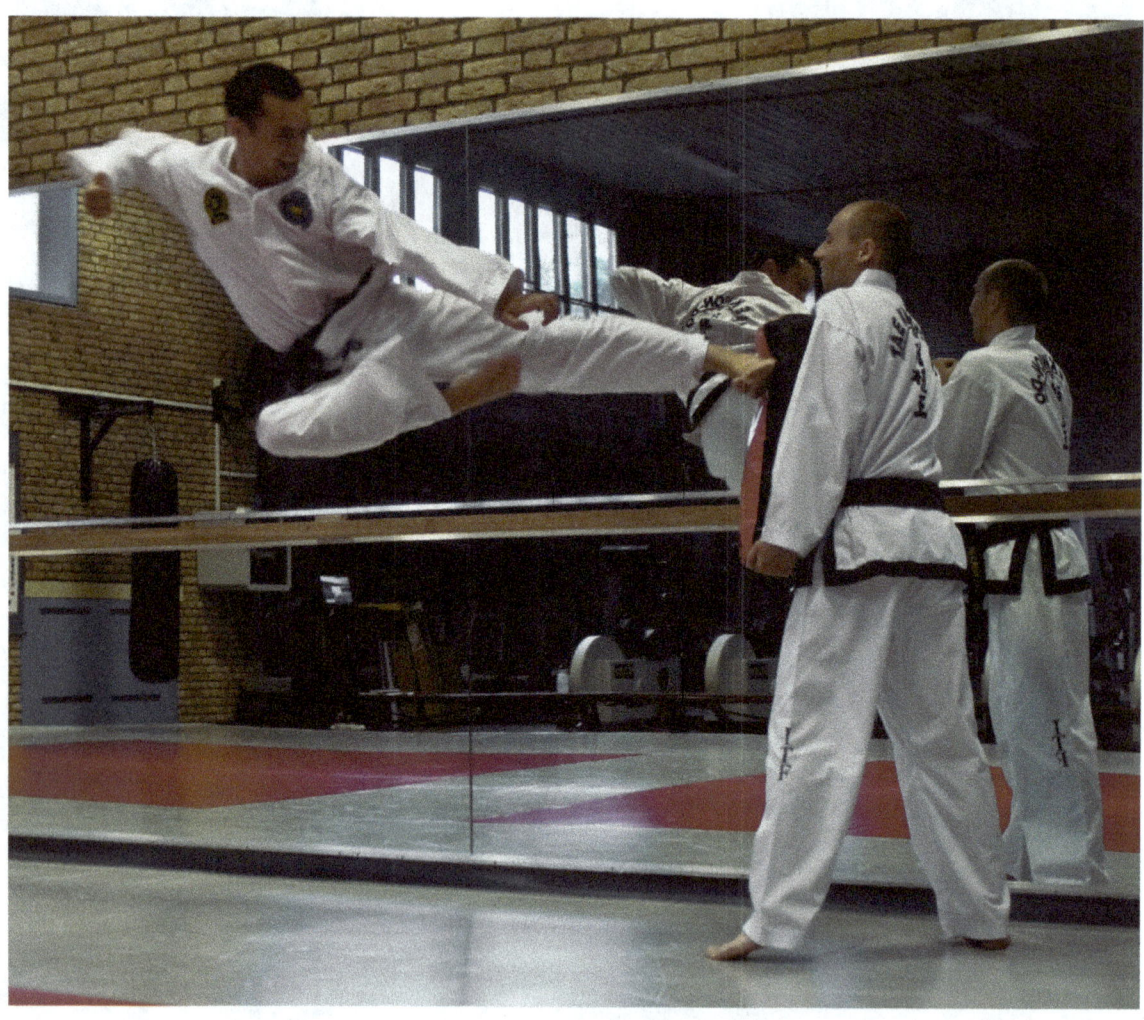

5. MENTAL ASPECTS OF TAEKWON-DO

Next to the exterior appearance, the origins of the martial art, and a manual for the physical aspects of Taekwon-Do have been described, there is still an important 'hidden' part. It is a part that everyone who practices Taekwon-Do experiences and that has motivated two people who practice Taekwon-Do to write this book. It is a part that is called 'Oriental' and is associated with 'Ki' or 'Chi'. Almost everyone knows or think they know what it is, but it is not very tangible. In this chapter the authors have tried to make a start in describing the mental aspect of Taekwon-Do. It is up to the student to interpret the material. It would not surprise the authors if, reading the book again many years from now, this interpretation has undergone major changes.

5.1 Chi

The body needs certain important things in order to function and stay alive. It needs energy to be able to fulfill daily tasks; think of nutrition, fluids, and sleep. Aside from these aspects, the body also possesses a different sort of energy, which is called *Chi* in Chinese. In Korean it is known as *Gi*, and in Japanese as *Ki*, but the Chinese name will be used since it is quite common.

Chi means 'life energy'. According to Eastern philosophy, the world consists of different elements; earth, water, fire, and air. This was shortly touched upon in Chapter 2. These elements 'radiate' a certain energy. Think of the warmth of the sun, a walk on the beach or in the forest; people often feel better after 'getting some fresh air'.

This life energy has a certain 'frequency'. The human body also has a certain frequency. For the majority of people, this frequency is different than that of the universe. Through exercises and meditation it is possible to decrease this difference or even reach a similar frequency as the universe. The advantage is that the body is enabled to make use of the energy that the universe has to offer. This energy can give strength, but it can also have a healing effect; it can take away physical or mental troubles.

For thousands of years, people have trained in using and adapting this energy. Many (Asian) martial arts are based on this principle: Tai *Chi* Chuan, Hap*ki*do, Ai*ki*do, etc. Chi also has an important role in medicine. In the Western world this is considered *alternative medicine*, but in East Asia this kind of medicine is in fact very common.

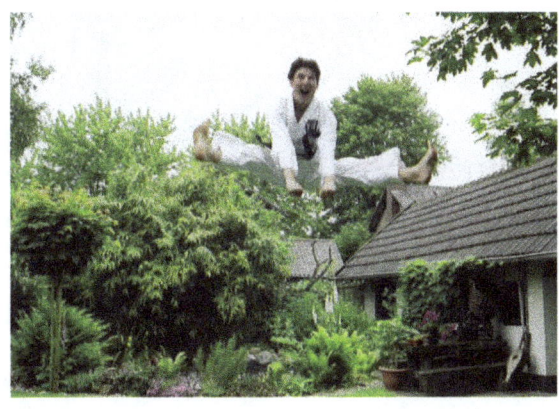

Twimyo Sangbal Ap Chagi.

5.2 Chakras

In the East, there are a number of basic principles that people live by. One of them is that there are certain energy fields in the body, also called chakras. There are seven main chakras:
- base chakra (located in the area between the anus and the genitalia);
- sacral chakra (in the upper part of the sacrum);
- solar plexus chakra (two finger widths above the bellybutton);
- heart chakra (the center of the chest);
- throat chakra (in the neck area);
- third eye chakra (in the center of the forehead);
- crown chakra (on the top of the head).

These chakras make sure certain parts of the body function well; every chakra has its own function. See Table 5.1 on the right.

Some stances (*Annun sogi*) and types of stretching in Taekwon-Do contribute to the development of the Chi. When the chakras are functioning properly, they will have a positive influence on the physical and mental development.

5.3 Meridians

Connected to the chakras are meridians (energy channels). These meridians run vertically through the entire body in order to transport the Chi to the right location. Sometimes, not enough Chi 'flows' through a meridian (because of stress, for example). When this is the case, one can break down these barriers with the help of meditation exercises and Chi exercises, which cause the Chi flow to course again and also cause some problems to disappear. This method is often used in acupuncture.

5.4 Vital parts (*Kupso*)

In line with the chakras and meridians, there are certain parts on the human body that are very vulnerable, which makes them ideal spots to direct an attack technique at. Some parts are vital, others only cause a temporary elimination. The body has hundreds of these vital spots. A number of them are known in some way, but most of them are 'secret' and only known to (Eastern) masters and practitioners of natural medicine. Next, the most well-known vital parts will be discussed.

For temporary elimination, one can think of:
- Nose;
- Eye socket;
- Jaw;
- Chin;
- Groin;
- Solar plexus.

With a punch or kick it is possible to temporarily eliminate someone by breaking their jaw or nose.

Some vital parts:
- Throat;
- Neck;
- Back.

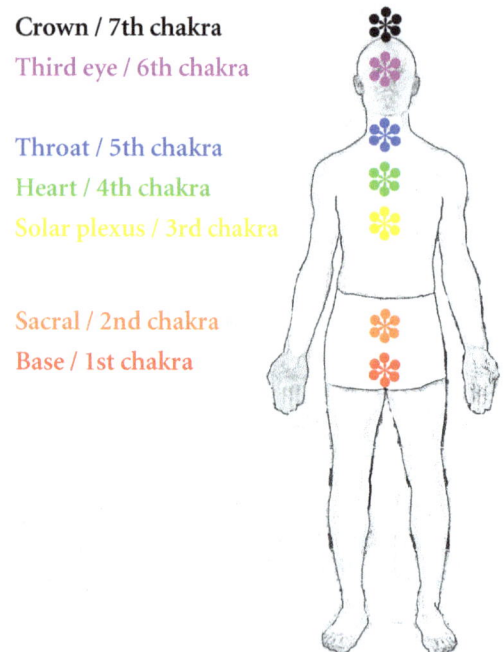

Crown / 7th chakra

Third eye / 6th chakra

Throat / 5th chakra

Heart / 4th chakra

Solar plexus / 3rd chakra

Sacral / 2nd chakra

Base / 1st chakra

	1st chakra (Base chakra)	2nd chakra (Sacral chakra)
Color/sense	Red, smell.	Orange, taste.
Relating to	Everything that is fixed, spine, bones, teeth, nails, both legs, anus, rectum, large intestine, back passage, prostate, blood.	Hip joint area, reproductive organs, kidneys, bladder, all fluids such as blood and sperm.
Development	Original life energy, primal self-confidence, connection to the earth and the material world, stability, and perseverance.	Original feelings, going with the flow of life, sensuality, eroticism, creativity, amazement, and enthusiasm.
	3rd chakra (Solar plexus chakra)	**4th chakra (Heart chakra)**
Color/sense	Yellow to golden yellow, seeing.	Green, touch.
Relating to	Lower back, abdominal cavity, digestive system, stomach, liver, spleen, gallbladder, and vegetative nervous system.	Upper back, heart, chest, lower part of the lungs, blood, blood circulation, skin, and hands.
Development	Character development, processing feelings and experiences, influence and power, strength and fullness, and wisdom.	Development of the heart, love, compassion, sharing with each other, selflessness, surrender, and healing.
	5th chakra (Throat chakra)	**6th chakra (Third eye chakra)**
Color/sense	Light blue, hearing.	Indigo, all senses, in the form of extrasensory perceptions as well.
Relating to	Upper part of the lungs, bronchi, esophagus, speech organs (voice), throat, neck, and jaws.	Cerebellum, ears, nose, sinuses, eyes, nervous system, forehead, and face.
Development	Communication, creative self-expression, openness, independence, and inspiration.	Awareness, intuition, development of the inner senses, mind power, projection of will, and manifestation.
	7th chakra (Crown chakra)	
Color/sense	Violet, white/connection to the cosmos.	
Relating to	Cerebrum, cranium.	
Development	Universal sense of being.	

Table 5.1 Function of the chakras

Sources: Brennan, Barbara Ann (2005).
Sharmon & Baginski (1990).

Significant parts of the body such as the major artery, windpipe, and nerves run through the neck/throat. When an attack technique is placed there, there is a chance that the person will be temporarily or even permanently eliminated. Because there are nerves running through the spinal column, the back is definitely a weak spot. One small fraction can lead to paralysis. This is why it is necessary for Taekwon-Do students to learn early on what the consequences of an attack are.

During partner and sparring exercises there is often a focus on these vital parts. All attack techniques are aimed at vital parts (determining the direction and position of a technique). Thrusting and striking techniques are mainly aimed at those parts of the body that are least protected, such as the neck, the throat, the solar plexus, and the eyes.

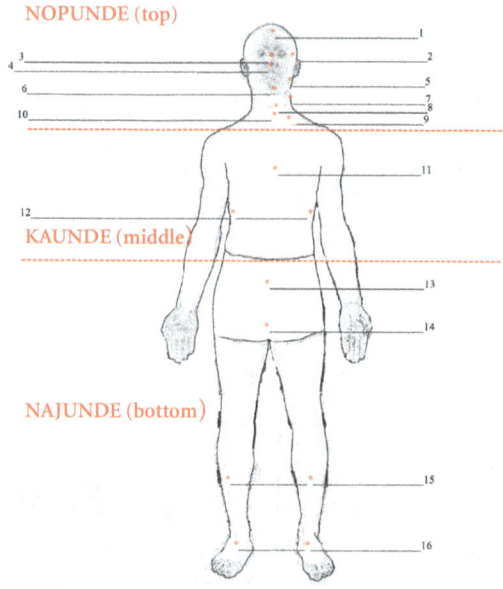

FRONT
1. Cranium, 2. Temple, 3. Nose (top), 4. Nose (bottom), 5. Jaw, 6. Chin, 7. Side of the neck, 8. Adam's apple, 9. Collarbone, 10. Trachea, 11. Solar plexus, 12. Floating ribs, 13. Abdomen, 14. Testicles, 15. Shins, 16. Upperside foot.

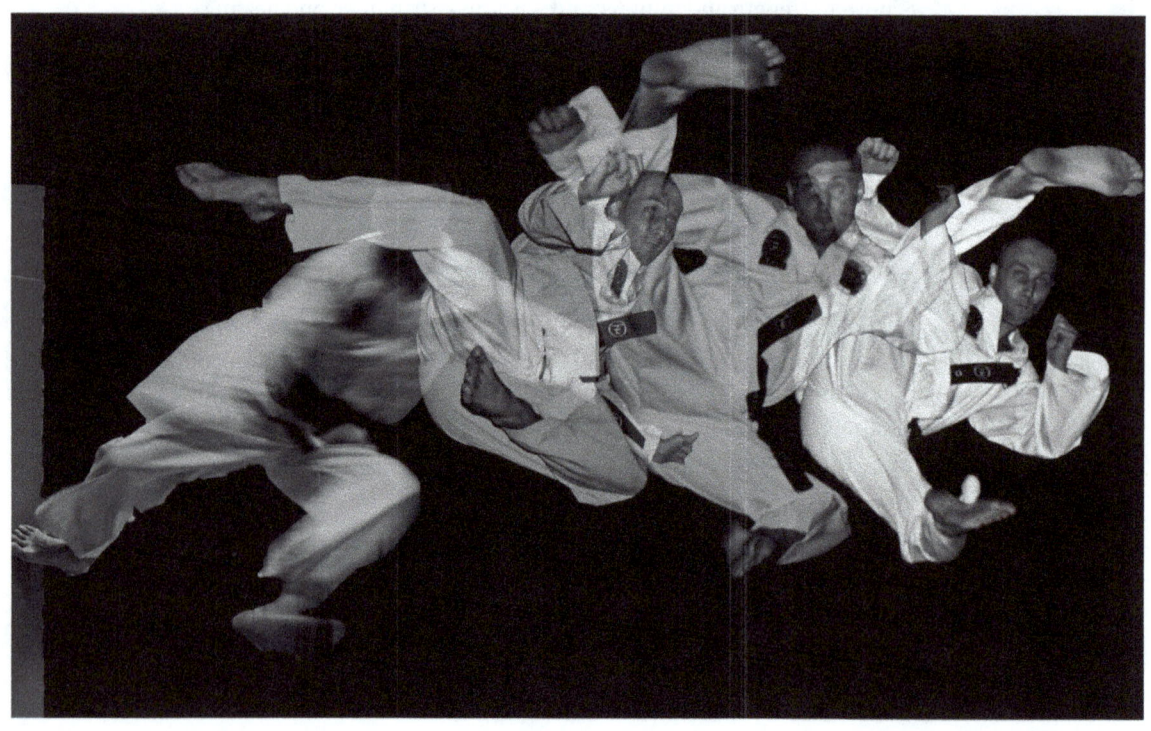

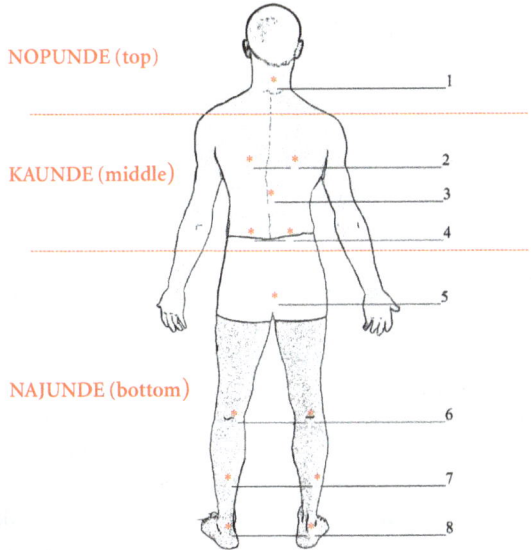

BACK
1. Skull base, 2. Shoulder-blades, 3. Spine, 4. Kidneys, 5. Coccyx, 6. Hollow of the knee, 7. Calf, 8. Achilles tendon.

5.5 Meditation (*Mong nyom*)

Scientific research often shows that the human brain is not fully utilized by far. Despite the fact that one is very conscious of some actions, there still are many things one does unconsciously. Thoughts are hard to control sometimes; many people suffer from concentration problems, fear of failure, or insecurity. By meditating it is possible to learn how to concentrate.

It is assumed that certain positions, such as the lotus position, activate certain chakras more. For the authors, the most important thing is that one assumes a position that feels comfortable. When this position is assumed, one tries to solely focus on one's in- and exhalation. However, slowly one will notice that the mind wanders and daily thoughts will enter the mind. When this happens, one should try to go back to focusing on breathing. This method will help to find peace and let go of any feelings of stress; it is ideal to perform before going to bed.

During meditation it is possible to visualize things. For example, one can imagine to be inhaling positive energy and exhaling negative energy. This method can also be performed when the body is in motion.

5. Mental aspects of Taekwon-Do

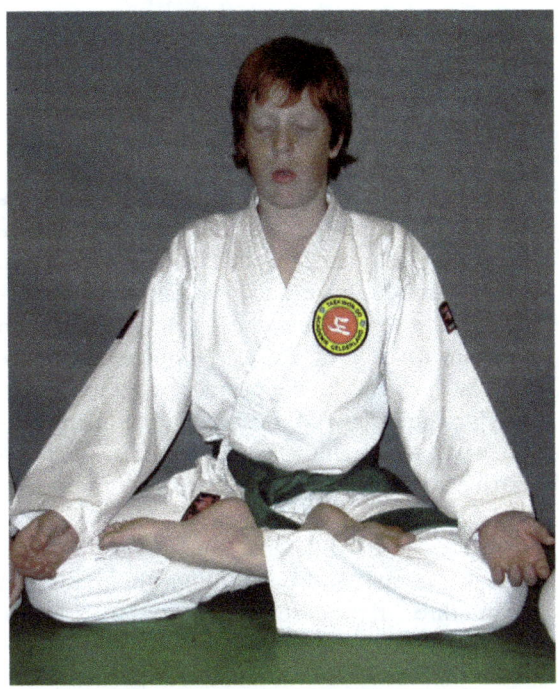

A young student of the authors in zen-meditation.

When performed regularly, there is a great chance that this method of meditation will have an effect on one's mental and physical wellbeing. Thoughts and inner strengths are often more powerful than is assumed.

5.6 Kihap

Kihaps play a significant part in Taekwon-Do. It is a scream or battle cry that can be let out during a technique with a great support of breath. Kihap literally means 'merging of energy'. Kihaps have been incorporated on fixed points in the *tuls* (see Part II for the tuls).

There are several reasons to use a kihap:

1. To support and give extra impact to a technique;
2. To forcefully contract the abdominal muscles, for the strength development of the technique, but also to protect the internal organs;

3. To gain self-confidence;
4. To frighten the opponent;
5 To focus even more on the technique;
6. To add a sense of entertainment.

In general, a kihap is used to add extra strength to a technique. However, it is also used to train resilience during a strike, punch, or kick from an opponent. This will subdue pain and possibly unconsciousness. One never inhales during an attack by an opponent or a block. An alert opponent will see when fatigue kicks in; the manner of breathing can easily give this away. Make sure the opponent cannot see this by training your breathing, during a sparring exercise for example.

There are several different ways of breathing: in through the nose and out through the mouth, in and out through the nose, or in and out through the mouth. The advantage of breathing in through the nose is that the air is heated and well purified, contrary to breathing in through the mouth. The advantage of breathing in through the mouth is that a lot of air comes in with one breath. Therefore, the amount of effort can influence the way one breathes.

The two basic ways to breathe are diaphragmatic breathing (from the stomach) and shallow breathing (from the chest).

With shallow breathing, the muscles between the ribs contract. Because of this contraction, the chest goes up and enlarges, and air is sucked into the lungs. With diaphragmatic breathing, the diaphragm is flexed, so that the chest cavity enlarges and air is sucked into the lungs. One will notice that the stomach slightly expands with diaphragmatic breathing. In a relaxed state, one usually uses diaphragmatic breathing. It is the form of breathing that takes up the least energy and has a relaxing effect. During strain, one often uses shallow breathing next to diaphragmatic breathing, since that is how the body is able to take up most oxygen.

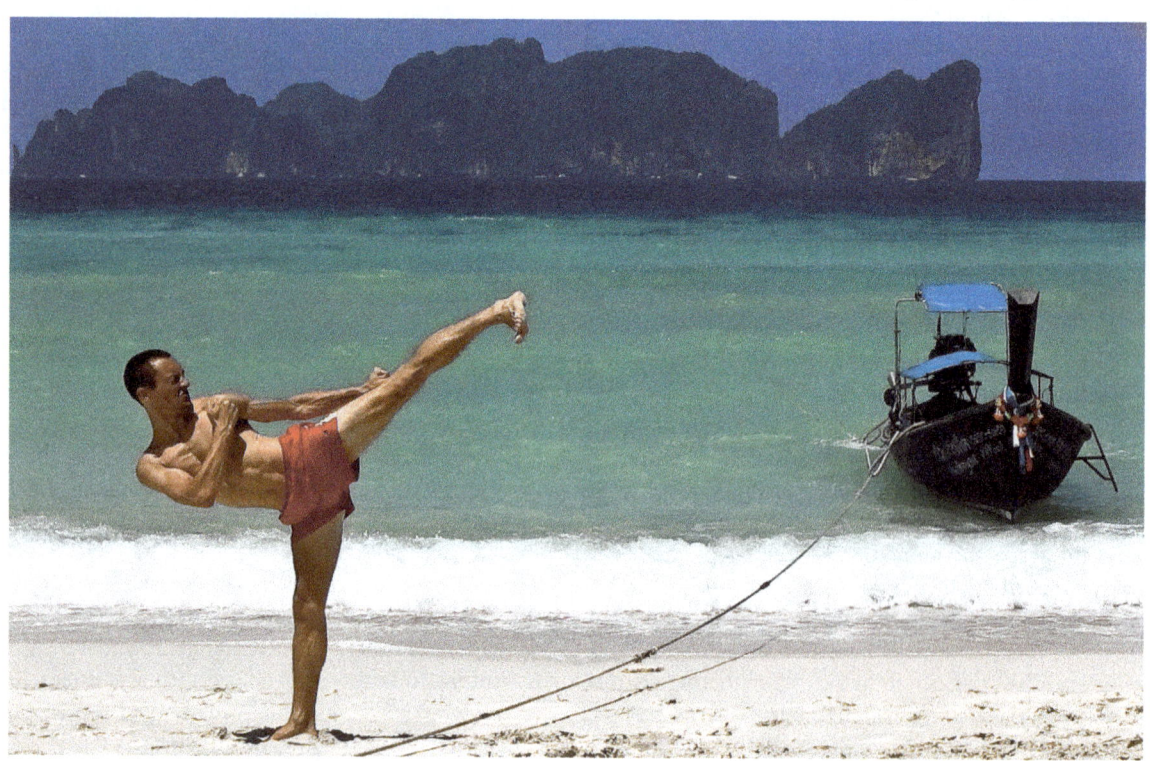

6. PRACTICAL TAEKWON-DO

In this chapter, the practical aspects of Taekwon-Do are discussed. This is a 'start' towards the next part of the book: Part II. This chapter deals with practical facets; from training materials to sparring techniques, and from exercises for beginners to exercises for the advanced students.

6.1 Training materials

Within Taekwon-Do, there are many different training materials to learn basic techniques or physical and mental skills. Next, a number of training materials is listed in a random order. There is an additional explanation for several of the materials. The Sabum, the instructor, can explain the use and training method of the following materials as well:

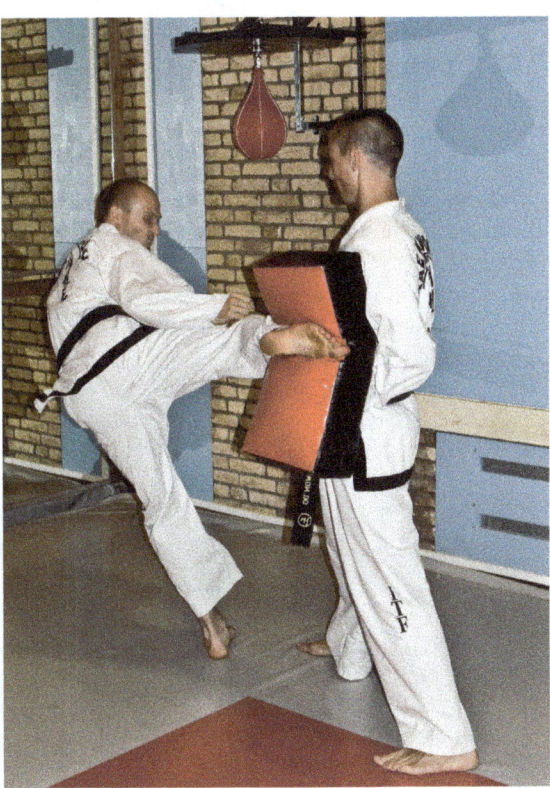

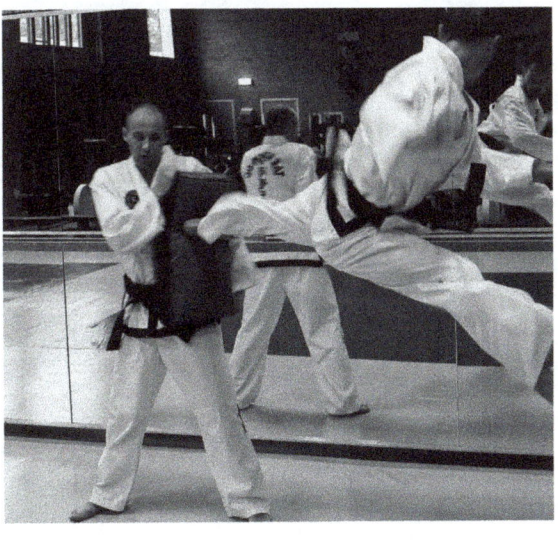

1. *Dan-Bong* (short stick);
2. *Jung-Bong* (middle stick);
3. *Dan-Geom* (knife);
4. Protectors (head, teeth, chest, hand, groin, shin, feet);
5. Jump rope;
6. Dumbells;
7. Ankle weights;
8. Jar;
9. Punching bag;
10. Hand pad/coaching mitt;

11. Hand mitt;
12. Punching bag (large-small);
13. Speedball;
14. *Dallyon Joo* (forging post);
15. Horizontal bar;
16. Mirror;
17. Boards (wood-synthetic material);
18. Holder for breaks.

Dallyon Joo ((forging post)

This is a post made of straw, rope, or similar material. The point of contact is hard; the post itself must lightly veer along with a punch or kick. Hands, arms, and feet are supposed to be hardened through striking, pushing, punching, or kicking techniques. Body parts are not meant to be injured. It is a perfect method to effectively train speed, strength, timing, precision, posture, controlled breathing, and concentration for a technique. Still, for the beginning student it takes courage and persistence to train with a Dallyon Joo.

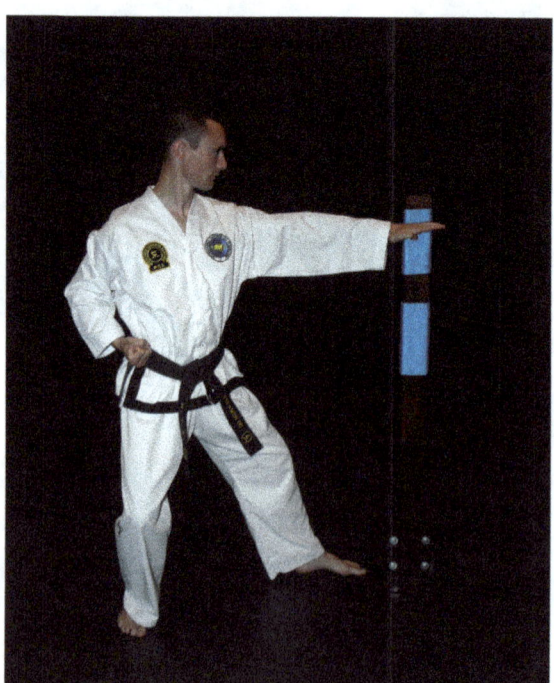

Speedball

The speedball is meant to train hand and foot techniques. Mostly, it is an effective training aid to train techniques for speed, precision, and timing, without a partner. Roundhouse kicks, twisting kicks, downward kicks, upward kicks, in- and outward kicks, are suitable to train on a speedball.

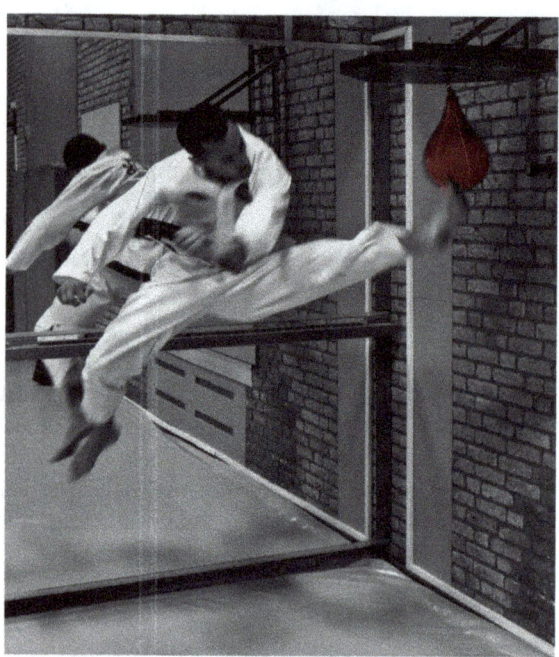

Hand mitt

The hand mitt is a very dynamic training aid. Since the person holding the hand mitt can very easily change positions, there are numerous ways to train. Explosiveness, speed, timing, and precision of different techniques can effectively be trained with a hand mitt. Also, the hand mitt is perfect for training techniques that want to go 'through the target'; think of a *Bandae Dollyo Goro Chagi* (reverse hooking kick).

Punching bag

In general, there are two types of punching bags; a big and a small bag. Usually the bags are filled with linen or grain. They are used to train hand and foot techniques. The larger or heavier bag has the most resistance and is therefore mostly used for strength development in techniques and endurance. The smaller bag is generally used for speed, precision, and timing. Punching bags are mostly used as fixed training materials, but they can also be used as dynamic training aids. By waving them around one creates a moving target, which makes timing and concentration very significant.

Mirror

Mirror training is an important part of Taekwon-Do. The mirror can be used to observe and correct one's own techniques. This way, techniques can be refined and what the authors call the 'proprioception' (sense of the position of body parts) can be increased. By using the mirror as a means of correction, one can become more skillful in techniques, and make it more powerful. For many students, the mirror is an incentive to practice step sparring (see Part II) at home without a partner, for example.

Alternatives

Not everyone has access to training materials all the time. This does not have to be a problem. There are many opportunities to optimally train without spending a lot of money. From old materials, it is fairly easy to make kicking bags, punching bags, and weights. There are also plenty of options to train outdoors. Think of e.g. tree trunks, dunes, and sandy plains. A serious Taekwon-Do student will make use of any opportunity to train.

6.2 Classification of techniques

Taekwon-Do techniques can be divided into two groups: primary techniques and secondary techniques. Next, the techniques will be presented in a diagram.

Main components	Subcomponents
1. General exercises	Warming up Stretching exercises Muscle strengthening exercises Endurance training Cooling down exercises
2. Fundamental exercises	Stances Walking techniques Hand techniques Foot techniques Jumping techniques Breathing exercises
3. Tuls	Chon-Ji (1st) 24 Tong-Il (24th)

4. Sparring	1-step
	2-step
	Foot technique sparring
	Semi-free sparring
	Sparring
	    Continuous system
	    Point-stop system
	    Other systems
	    Multiple opponents

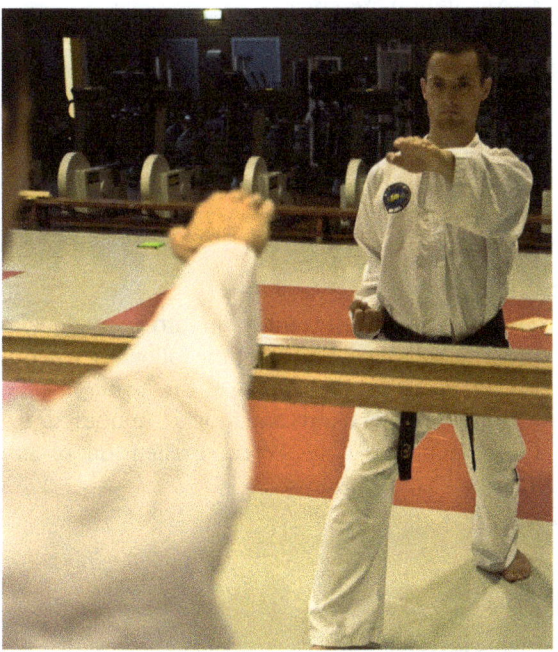

Main components	Subcomponents
5. Break tests	Hand techniques Foot techniques Jumping techniques Combination techniques
6. Special techniques	Demonstration exercises Muscle control
7. Self-defense	Self-defense techniques Control techniques Throwing techniques Weapon defense Breaking a fall
8. Esoteric exercises	Strength development exercises Meditative exercises Concentration exercises Mental exercises

In this paragraph, the different hand and foot techniques have been arranged, and the body parts with which one hits the target have been documented. In Taekwon-Do, every technique has a specific body part with which one performs the technique. Accordingly, every technique has one or more (vital) targets.

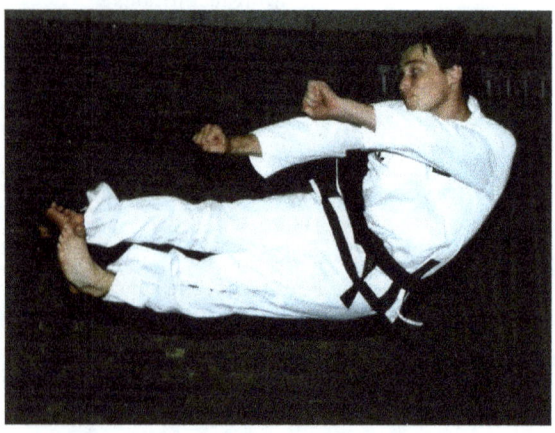

Twimyo Sangbal Yopcha Jirugi.

For example, the fist punch is made with the knuckles of the index finger and middle finger. The punch can be directed at the solar plexus or jaw, but is not meant for the elbow, for instance. A technique with the side of the fist is suitable for the elbow.

Every technique has its own objective. A strike is often meant to break something, a thrust has the goal to puncture something like a knife, and a punch has an intense effect. This often causes a punch to inflict internal damage. The basic techniques will be explained in the exercise book.

There is a relationship between techniques and targets, and this relationship is based on science. When the student knows this relationship and can perform the techniques in a technically correct manner, a relatively small effort can have the desired results.

Arrangement of techniques into categories
Taekwon-Do has many techniques or skills, such as:

- Stances;
- Breathing exercises;
- Meditation exercises;
- Forms of walking;
- Blocks;
- Freeing techniques;
- Controlling techniques;
- Defensive techniques;
- Attack techniques;
- Breaking falls;
- Floor techniques.

The authors do not want to go into every detail of these techniques. The goal of the following schedule is to give a general overview of the *arrangement* of the fundamental hand- and foot techniques, so that the student has a better comprehension of how Taekwon-Do is composed.

Right page: Figure 6.1 Overview of techniques

6. Practical Taekwon-Do

Hand techniques (*soo gi*)		Foot techniques (*jok gi*)	
Defensive technique (*Bang Eo Gi*)	Attack technique (*Gong Gyuk Gi*)	Defensive technique (*Bang Eo Gi*)	Attack technique (*Gong Gyuk Gi*)
Blocks:	**Punches:**	**Blocks:**	**Kicks:**
• Low Block (*Najunde Makgi*) • Middle Block (*Kaunde Makgi*) • High Block (*Nopunde Makgi*) • Horizontal Block (*Soopyong Makgi*) • W-shape Block (*San Makgi*) • U-shape Block (*Digutja Makgi*) • Circular Block (*Dollimyo Makgi*) • Double Arc Hand Block (*Doo Bandalson Makgi*) • Twin Forearm Block (*Sang Palmok Makgi*) • Guarding Block (*Daebi Makgi*) • Scooping Block (*Duro Makgi*) • Louring Block (*Yuin Makgi*) • Pushing Block (*Miro Makgi*) • Parallel Block (*Narani Makgi*) • Grasping Block (*Butjaba Makgi*) • Hooking Block (*Golcho Makgi*) • Pressing Block (*Noollo Makgi*) • Downward Block (*Naeryo Makgi*)	• Walking Stance Obverse Punch (*Gunnun So Baro Jirugi*) • Walking Stance Reverse Punch (*Gunnun So Bandae Jirugi*) • L-stance Obverse Punch (*Niunja So Baro Jirugi*) • L-stance Reverse Punch (*Niunja So Bandae Jirugi*) • Rear Foot Stance Obverse Punch (*Dwitbal So Baro Jirugi*) • Rear Foot Stance Reverse Punch (*Dwitbal So Bandae Jirugi*) • Vertical Stance Punch (*Soojik So Jirugi*) • X-stance Punch (*Kyocha So Jirugi*) • Twin Fist Punch (*Sang Joomuk Jirugi*) • Vertical Punch (*Sewo Jirugi*) • Upward Punch (*Ollyo Jirugi*) • Upset Punch (*Dwijibun Jirugi*) • U-shape Punch (*Digutja Jirugi*)	• Front Upward Kick (*Apcha Ollyo*) • Side Upward Kick (*Yopcha Ollyo*) • Crescent Kick (*Bandal Chagi*) • Waving Kick (*Doro Chagi*) • Checking Kick (*Cha Momchugi*) • Side Checking Kick (*Yopcha Momchugi*) • Front Checking Kick (*Apcha Momchugi*) • Hooking Kick (*Golcho Chagi*)	• Side Piercing Kick (*Yopcha Jirugi*) • Back Piercing Kick (*Dwitcha Jirugi*) • Back Pushing Kick (*Dwitcha Milgi*) • Side Thrusting Kick (*Yopcha Tulgi*) • Side Pushing Kick (*Yopcha Milgi*) • Front Snap Kick (*Apcha Busugi*) • Side Front Snap Kick (*Yopap Cha Busugi*) • Back Snap Kick (*Dwitcha Busugi*) • Stamping Kick (*Bap Chagi*) • Turning Kick (*Dollyo Chagi*) • Side Turning Kick (*Yop Dollyo Chagi*) • Downward Kick (*Naeryo Chagi*) • Pick-shape Kick (*Gok-Kaeng-I-Chagi*) • Upward Kick (*Ollyo Chagi*) • Reverse Turning Kick (*Bandae Dollyo Chagi*) • Reverse Hooking Kick (*Bandae Dollyo Goro Chagi*) • Twisting Kick (*Bituro Chagi*) • Vertical Kick (*Sewo Chagi*)

Hand techniques (*soo gi*)		Foot techniques (*jok gi*)	
- Upward Block (*Ollyo Makgi*) - Rising Block (*Chookyo Makgi*) - Checking Block (*Momchau Makgi*) - Double Forearm Block (*Doo Palmok Makgi*) - Side Front Block (*Yopap Makgi*) - Side Block (*Yop Makgi*) - Front Block (*Ap Makgi*) - Outward Block (*Bakuro Makgi*)	- Downward Punch (*Naeryo Jirugi*) - Crescent Punch (*Bandal Jirugi*) - Turning Punch (*Dollyo Jirugi*) - Angle Punch (*Giokja Jirugi*) - Knuckle Fist Punch (*Sonkarak Joomuk Jirugi*) - Horizontal Punch (*Soopyong Jirugi*) - Long Fist Punch (*Ghin Joomuk Jirugi*) - Open Fist Punch (*Pyon Joomuk Jirugi*) - Double Fist Punch (*Doo Joomuk Jirugi*)	- Pressing Kick (*Noollo Chagi*) - Sweeping Kick (*Suroh Chagi*) - Grasping Kick (*Butjabo Chagi*) - Straight Kick (*Jigeau Chagi*) - Foot Tackling (*Bal Golgi*) - Slip Kick (*Durokamyo Chagi*)	
	Strikes: - Upper Elbow Strike (*Wi Palkup Taerigi*) - Upper Back Elbow Strike (*Widwi Palkup Taerigi*) - High Elbow Strike (*Nopun Palkup Taerigi*) - Inward Strike (*Anuro Taerigi*) - Downward Strike (*Naeryo Taerigi*) - Outward Strike (*Bakuro Taerigi*) - Side Strike (*Yop Taerigi*) - Horizontal Strike (*Soopyong Taerigi*) - Front Strike (*Ap Taerigi*)	**Flying kicks:** - Flying Front Kick (*Twimyo Ap Chagi*) - Flying Turning Kick (*Twimyo Dollyo Chagi*) - Flying Reverse Turning Kick (*Twimyo Bandae Dollyo Chagi*) - Flying Side Piercing Kick (*Twimyo Yopcha Jirugi*) - Flying Side Thrusting Kick (*Twimyo Yopcha Tulgi*) - Flying Side Pushing Kick (*Twimyo Yopcha Milgi*) - Flying Back Kick (*Twimyo Dwit Chagi*) - Flying Twisting Kick (*Twimyo Bituro Chagi*) - Flying Vertical Kick (*Twimyo Sewo Chagi*)	

6. Practical Taekwon-Do

Hand techniques (*soo gi*)	Foot techniques (*jok gi*)
- Crescent Strike *(Bandal Taerigi)* - Backside Strike *(Yopdwi Taerigi)* - Side Front Strike *(Yopap Taerigi)* **Thrusts:** - Downward Thrust *(Naeryo Tulgi)* Straight Fingertip Thrust *(Sun Sonkut Tulgi)* - Upset Fingertip Thrust *(Dwijibun Sonkut Tulgi)* - Twin Side Elbow Thrust *(Sang Yop Palkup Tulgi)* - Side Front Thrust *(Yopap Tulgi)* - Horizontal Thrust *(Soopyong Tulgi)* **Cuts:** - Outward Cross Cut *(Bakuro Ghutgi)* - Inward Cross Cut *(Anuro Ghutgi)* - Side Cross Cut *(Yop Ghutgi)*	- Overhead Kick *(Twio Nomo Chagi)* - Flying Downward Kick *(Twimyo Naeryo Chagi)* - Flying Twin Foot Front Kick *(Twimyo Sangbal Ap Chagi)* - Flying Twin Foot Side Piercing Kick *(Twimyo Sangbal Yopcha Jirugi)* - Flying Double Foot Side Pushing Kick *(Twimyo Doobal Yopcha Milgi)* - Flying Twin Foot Turning Kick *(Twimyo Sangbal Dollyo Chagi)* - Flying Twin Foot Twisting Kick *(Twimyo Sangbal Bituro Chagi)* - Flying Scissors-shape Kick *(Twimyo Kawi Chagi)* - Flying Crescent Kick *(Twimyo Bandal Chagi)* - Flying Two Directional Kick *(Twimyo Sangbal Chagi)* - Flying Spiral Kick *(Twimyo Rasonsik Chagi)*

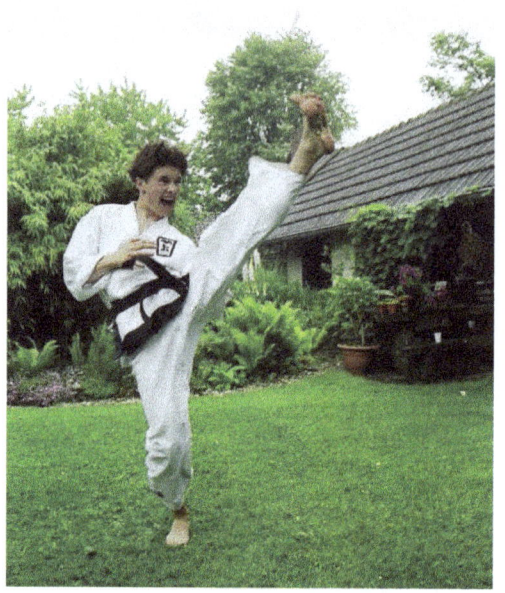

Yop Apcha Ollyo Busugi.

Striking surfaces

Next, the body parts with which one hits the target are presented in text and image.

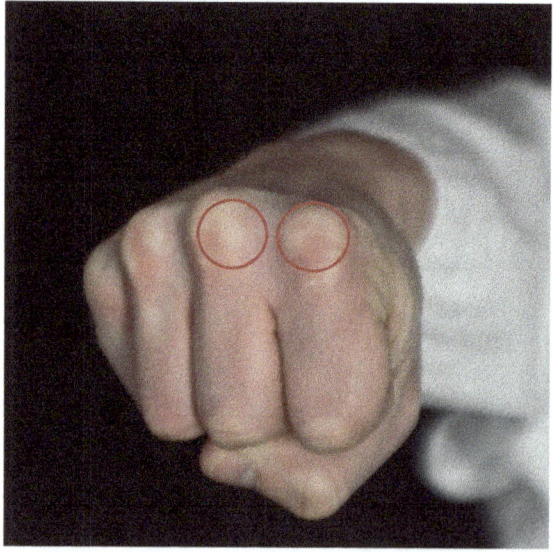

FOREFIST *(Ap Joomuk)*

The knuckles of the index- and middle fingers are the striking surface. The knuckles must be in line with the underarm, while the thumb is underneath. The wrist must not be bent and the fist must be completely closed at the moment of the strike, so that there is no room in between the fingers. This attack technique can be directed at the stomach, ribs, jaw, etc. Also, the fore fist is used for several blocks.

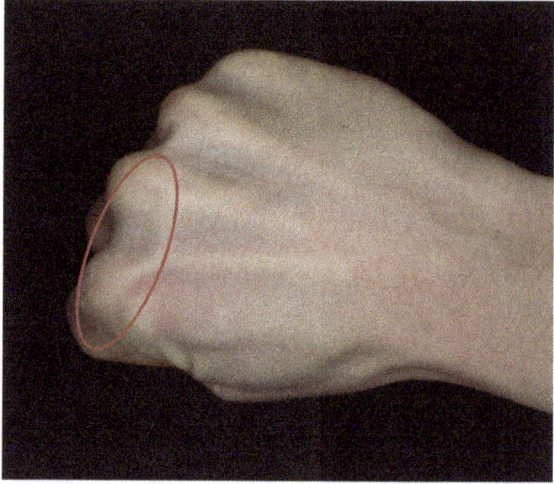

BACK FIST *(Dung Joomuk)*

The knuckles of the index and middle fingers are the striking surface. This attack technique can be directed at the temple, skull, ribcage, or stomach.

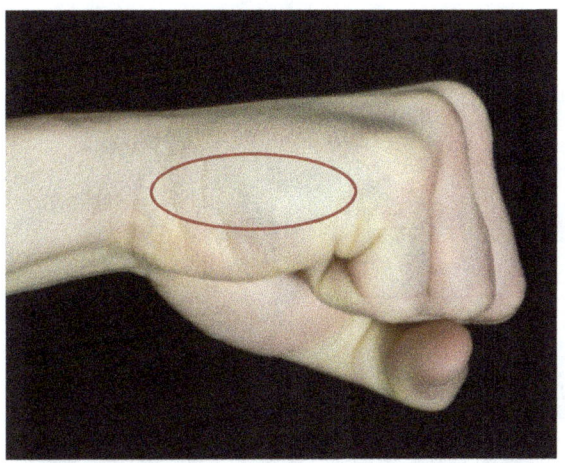

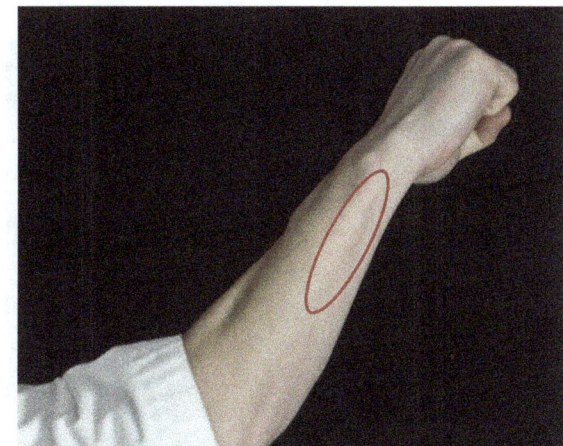

SIDE FIST *(Yop Joomuk)*

This technique can be used for an attack toward the skull, breastbone, upper lip, stomach, or ribs. With some countermovements the side fist points towards one's own body part.

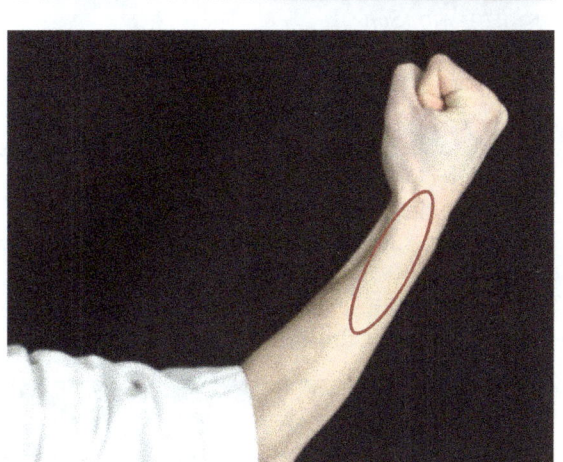

FOREARM *(Palmok)*

This body part is used for blocking. One blocks with about one third of the arm (from wrist to elbow). The forearm can be divided into the outside forearm (side of the pinky) and the inside forearm (side of the thumb).

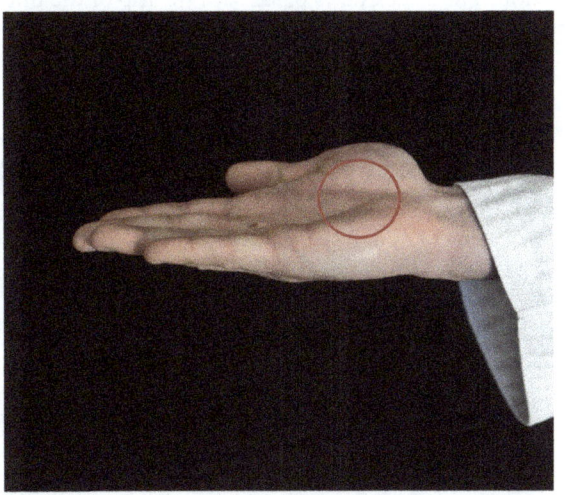

PALM *(Sonbadak)*

The fingers are slightly bent in order to make the palm more solid. Make sure the thumb is next to the hand. This part is mainly used for blocks. In some cases, this technique is used to place an attack on e.g. the face.

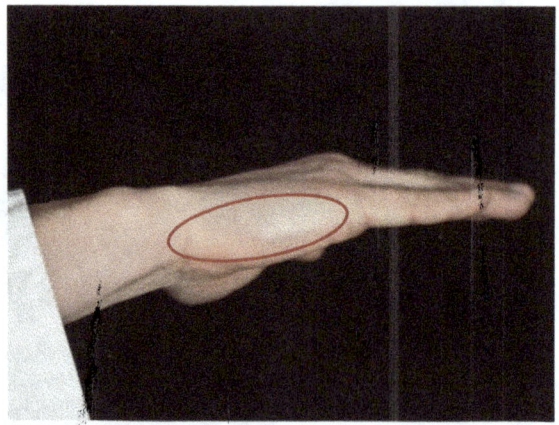

KNIFE HAND *(Sonkal)*

This part of the hand is mainly used as an attack technique directed at the neck, nose, shoulder, or ribs. Also, the knife hand is ideal as a block. The advantage of blocking with the knife hand is that one can quickly switch to grabbing the opponent or the object of attack. Make sure that when making a knife hand, the fingers are slightly bent, firm next to each other with a little bit of space between the thumb and index finger.

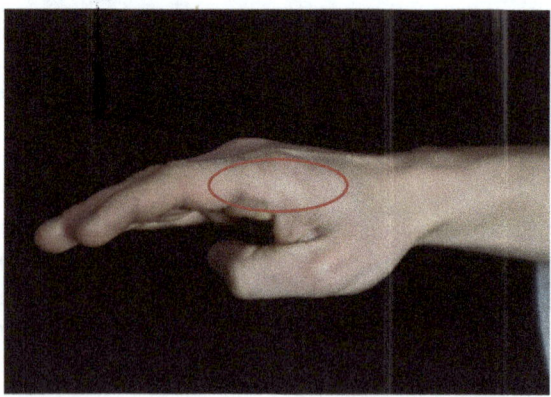

INNER KNIFE HAND *(Sonkal Dung)*

The inner knife hand is generally the same as the knife hand. Make sure that the thumb is retracted, facing the palm. It is possible to place an attack with the side of the knuckle of the index finger. This attack technique can be directed at the neck, nose, chin, temple, or ribs. It is also used as a block.

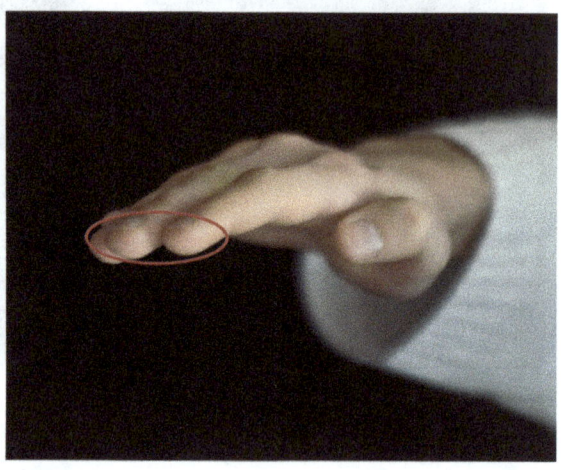

FINGERTIPS *(Sonkut)*

This part of the hand has to be treated with precision. The attack takes place with the top of the middle, index, and ring finger. The technique is mostly aimed at soft targets. Think of the throat, eyes, solar plexus, armpits, and pubic bone.

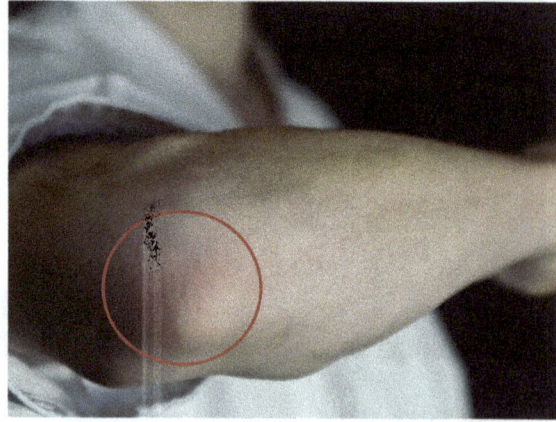

ELBOW *(Palkup)*

An attack with the elbow can be quite destructive. It is an ideal technique to use when the distance between you and the opponent is small. Several possible targets are the chin, jaw, chest and stomach.

6. Practical Taekwon-Do

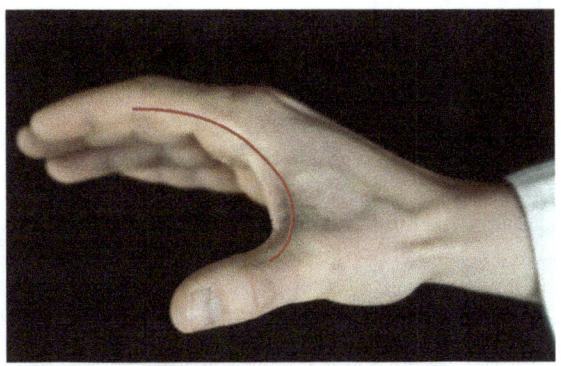

Arc hand *(Bandal Son)*

The index finger is slightly bent while the other fingers are bent deeper. The thumb deviates in the direction of the little finger. The space between the second knuckle of the index finger and the thumb is used for blocks, holds, and attacks. E.g. the neck, Adam's apple, or tip of the chin can be attacked.

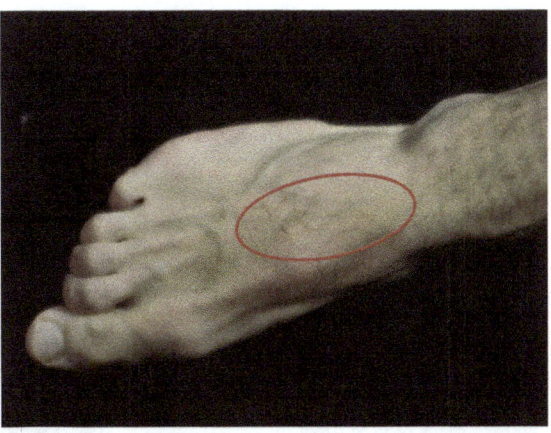

Instep *(Baldung)*

The advantage of kicking with the instep instead of the ball of the foot is that a greater distance is created by stretching the ankle joint and bending the toes away from the body a little. The disadvantage is that the foot is more vulnerable at the moment of the attack. The possible targets are similar to those of the ball of the foot.

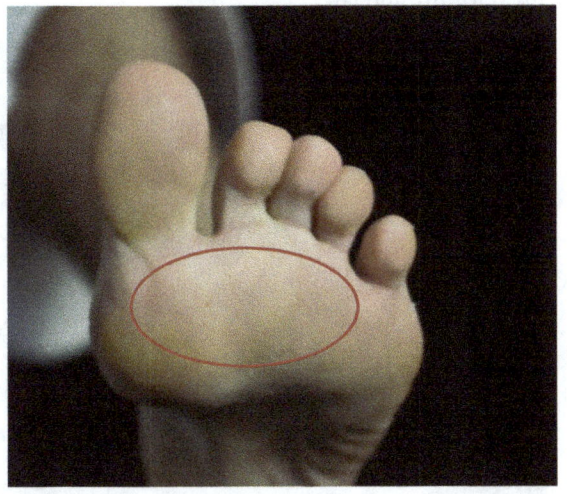

Ball of the foot *(Apkumchi)*

This part of the foot is often used when performing a round or front kick towards the entire face, ribs, solar plexus, stomach, chest, or groin. By stretching the toes well, the ball of the foot will be available to use.

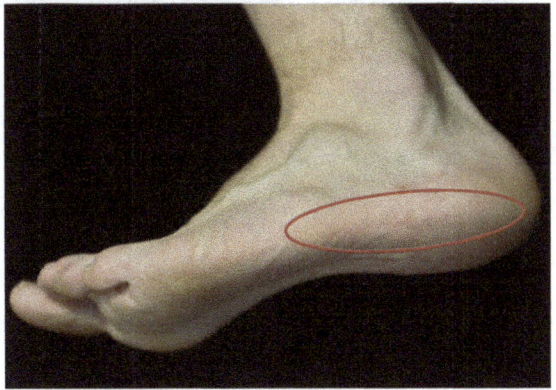

Foot sword *(Balkal)*

One third of the edge (sword) of the foot is used. This part of the foot must be in line with the bottom part of the leg. The foot sword needs to be pointed towards the target whereas the toes point downward towards the own leg. This technique can serve as an attack on the armpit, ribcage, knee, bridge of the nose, neck, etc.

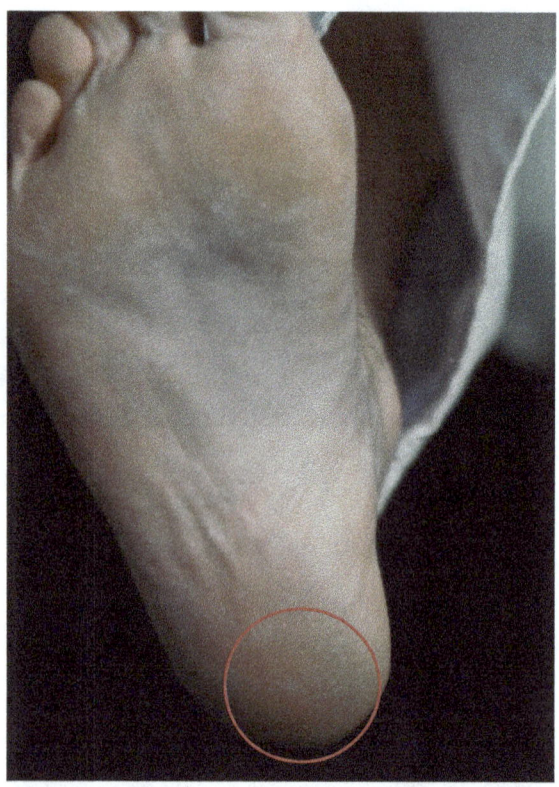

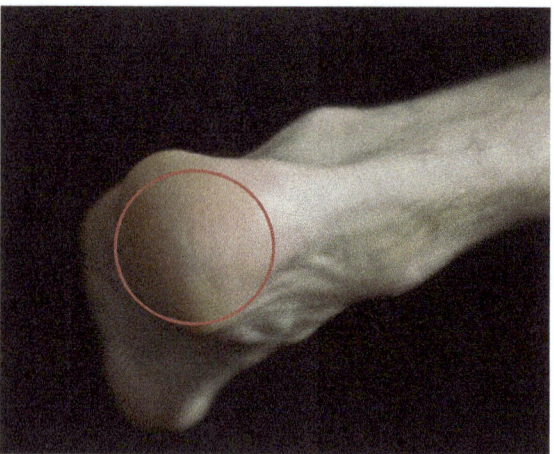

BACK HEEL *(Dwichook)*

One kicks with the backside of the heel; the bone underneath the Achilles tendon. This attack technique can be used for the temple, breastbone, upper lip, scrotum, and jaw.

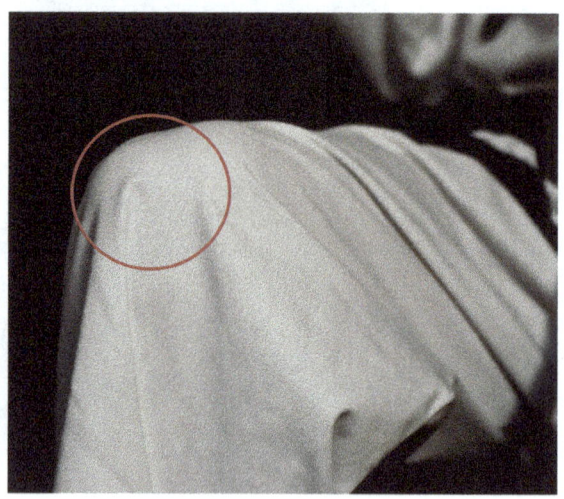

BACK SOLE *(Dwitkumchi)*

This is the bottom of the heel. This part is often used to attack in a stomping manner. The metatarsal is one of the possible targets.

KNEE *(Moorup)*

The knee is used when there is a short fighting distance. This attack technique can be directed at the face, breastbone, ribcage, stomach, or scrotum.

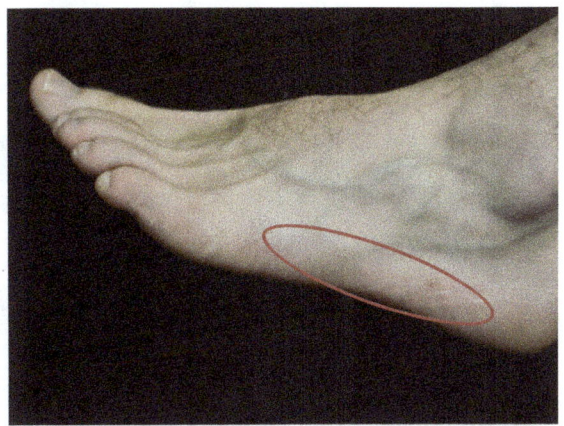

SIDE INSTEP *(Yop Baldung)*

The ankle is strongly bent upward and twisted outward. The instep of the foot arrives almost downward on the target. This technique is mainly used for blocks on for example the underarm or shin.

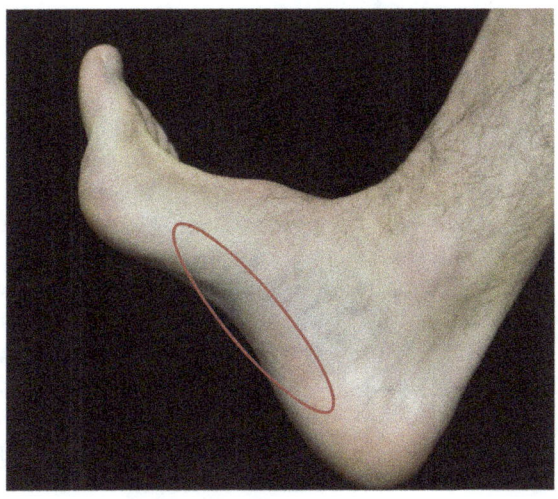

REVERSE FOOT SWORD *(Balkal Dung)*

The ankle and toes are bent. This technique can be used at an angle of 90 degrees to be directed at the face, chest, or breastbone.

Remaining striking surfaces
There are other surfaces to attack or block a target with. One can think of the toes, shin, calf, extended fist, open fist, one or two fingers, thumb, middle knuckles, bent wrist, bear hand, shoulders, back of the head, and forehead.

6.3 Stances (*Sogi*)

There are many different stances within Taekwon-Do. A correct stance is of great importance; it helps one to get the most out of an attack or defense. Next to being a requisite for a good technical execution, the stance has other goals. Think of balance and strength training, but also of the stance as a philosophical value (see *tuls*, Chapter 7.2). During the training, one will notice that some techniques are easier to perform depending on the chosen stance. Next, the stances that one encounters on the way to the 1st dan are described. The illustrated feet show how big the stance must be and from which body part it is measured.

Attention Stance *(Charyot Sogi)*
This stance has been discussed in Paragraph 1.3; the greeting procedure.

Parallel Stance *(Narani Sogi)*
One stands one shoulder width wide, toes pointing forward.

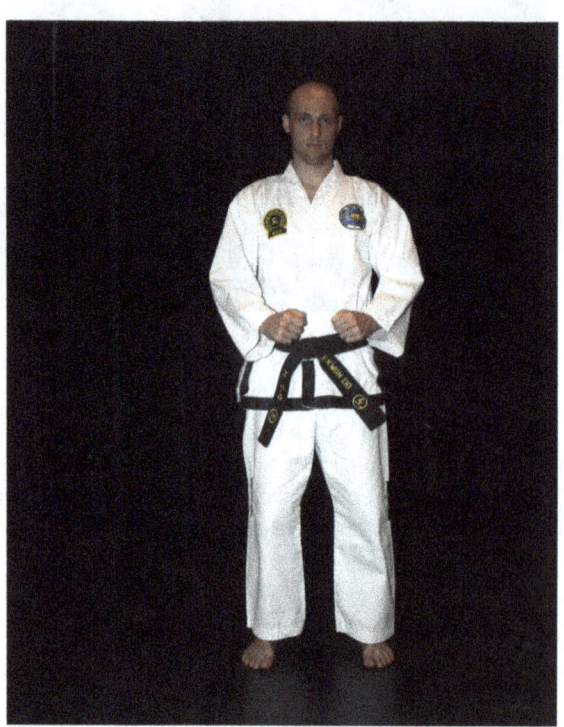

NARANI SOGI
One shoulder width

Closed Stance *(Moa Sogi)*
The feet are together with no space in between.

Walking Stance *(Gunnun Sogi)*
One stands one shoulder width wide, and one and a half shoulder width long. With the walking stance, pay attention to these aspects:

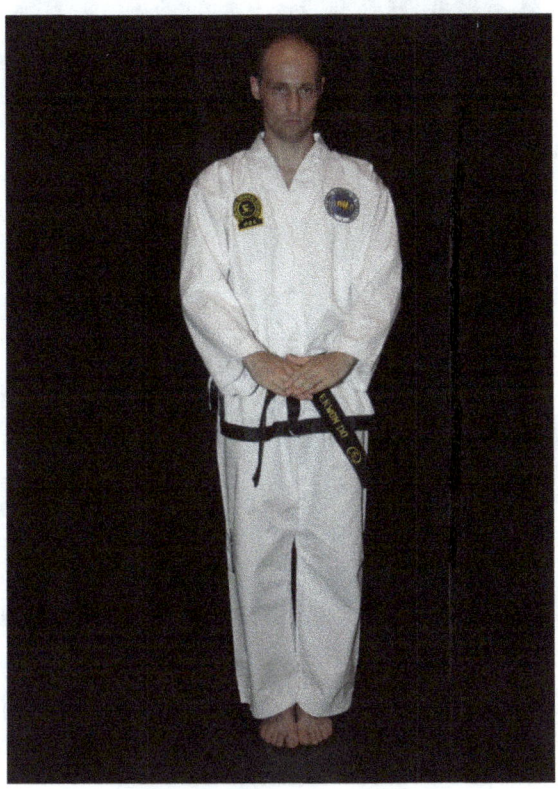

MOA SOGI

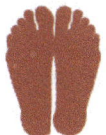

GUNNUN SOGI
One shoulder width wide
One and a half shoulder width from toe to toe

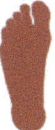

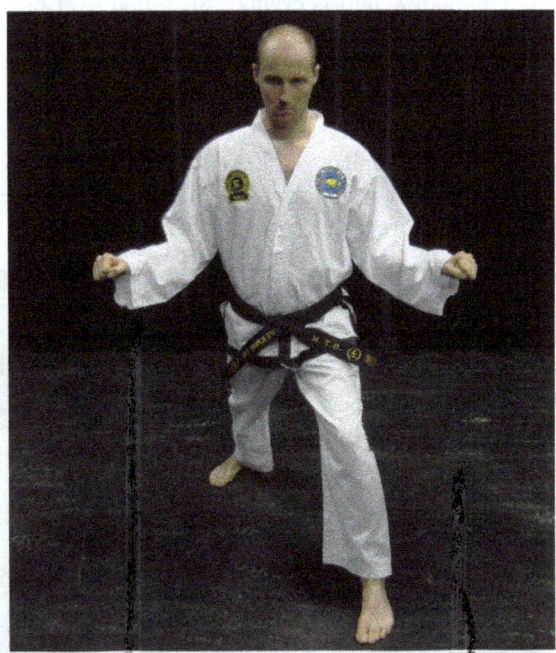

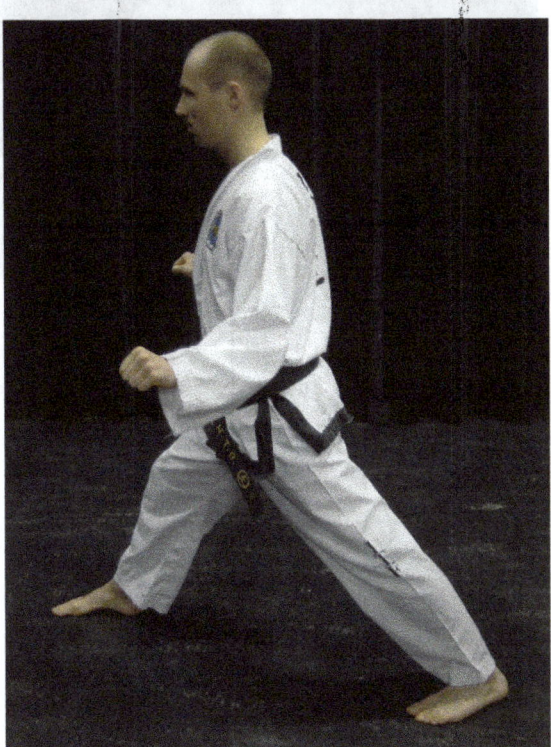

1. The front leg is bent, the kneecap must be in line with the heel. The toes must point forward.
2. The rear leg must be stretched, toes pointing outward by approximately 25 degrees.
3. The bodyweight is evenly distributed over both legs. This offers the opportunity to easily perform a technique with either leg.

Low Stance *(Nachuo Sogi)*
This stance is similar to the walking stance, with the exception that it is about one foot length longer. This gives more length in an attack technique.

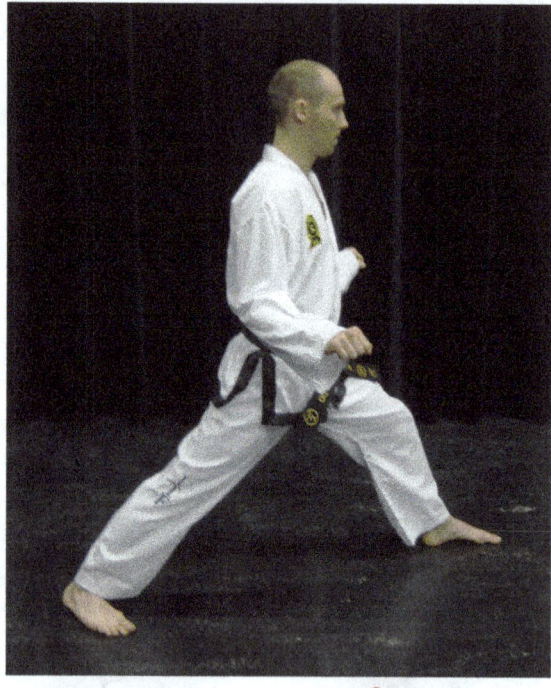

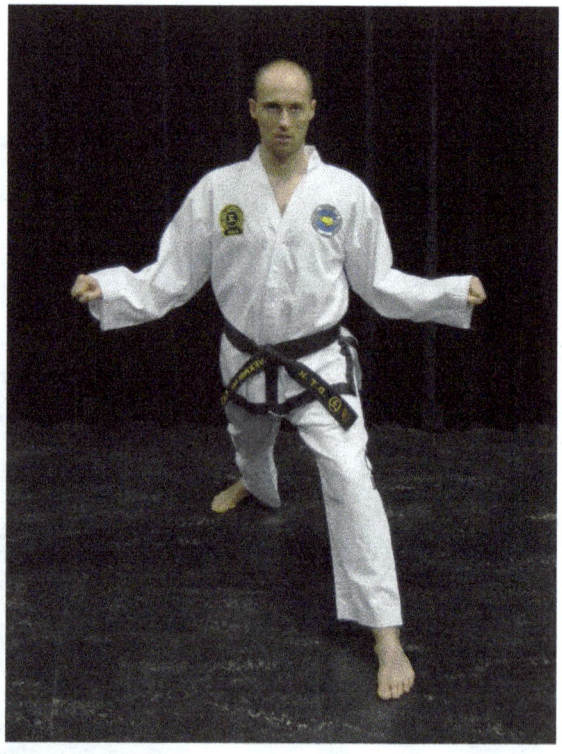

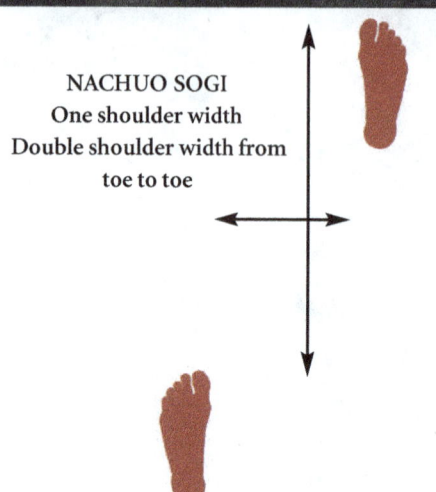

NACHUO SOGI
One shoulder width
Double shoulder width from toe to toe

L-Stance *(Niunja Sogi)*
The length is one and a half shoulder widths, both toes point slightly inward for more stability. Attention points with the L-stance are:

1. Both knees are bent.
2. The knee of the rear leg must be in a vertical line with the toes.
3. The rear leg must carry 70% of the bodyweight, while the front leg carries 30%. This creates the opportunity to easily perform a technique with the front leg.

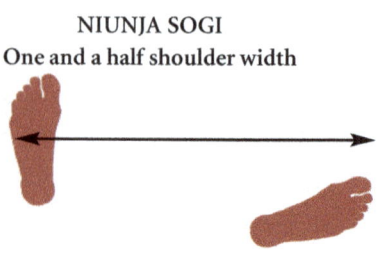

NIUNJA SOGI
One and a half shoulder width

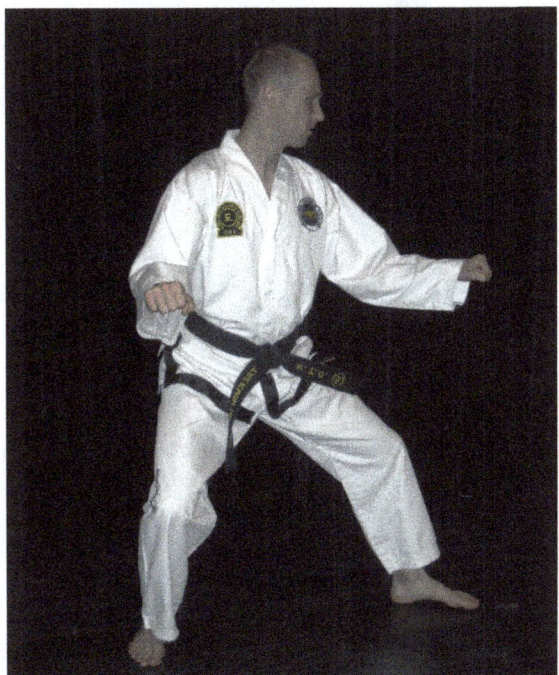

This is a suitable stance for making backwards kicks, such as a *Dwit Chagi*.

Fixed Stance *(Gojung Sogi)*
This stance is similar to the L-stance; the only difference is that it is half a foot length longer and that the bodyweight is evenly distributed over both legs. This creates more length during the attack technique.

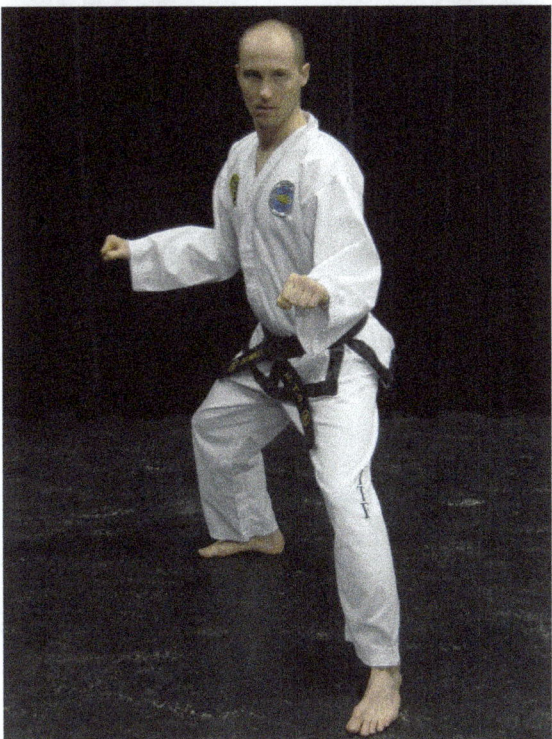

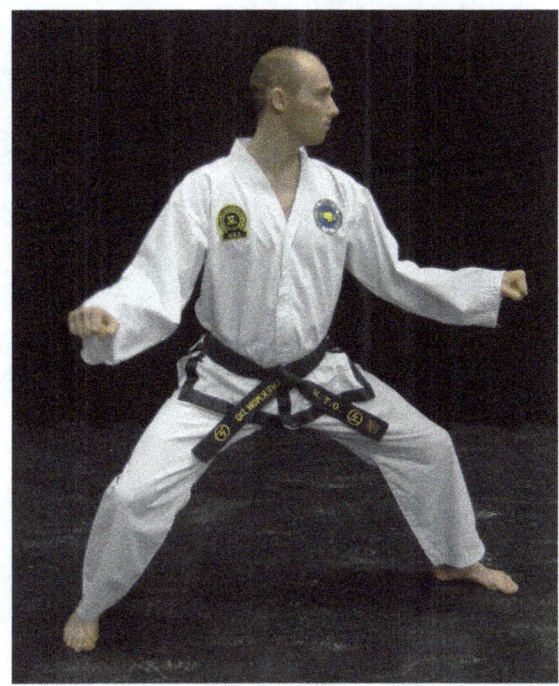

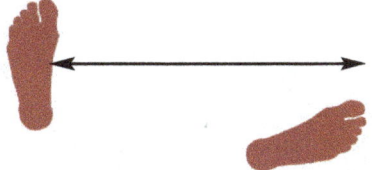

GOJUNG SOGI
One and a half shoulder width

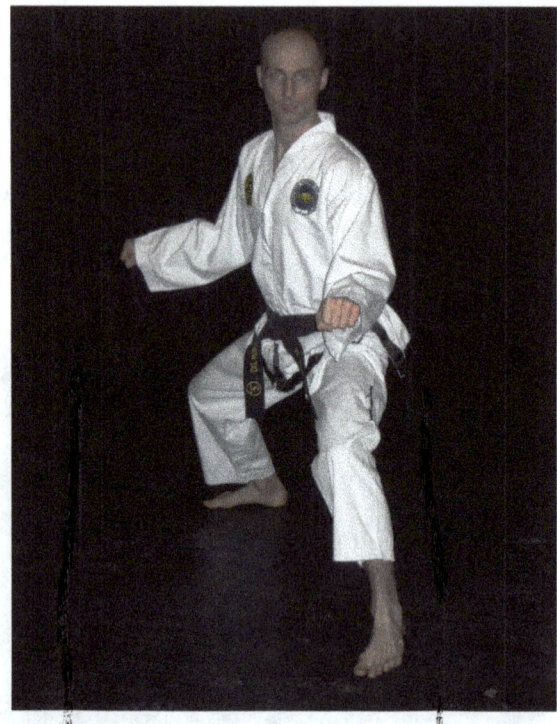

Sitting Stance *(Annun Sogi)*

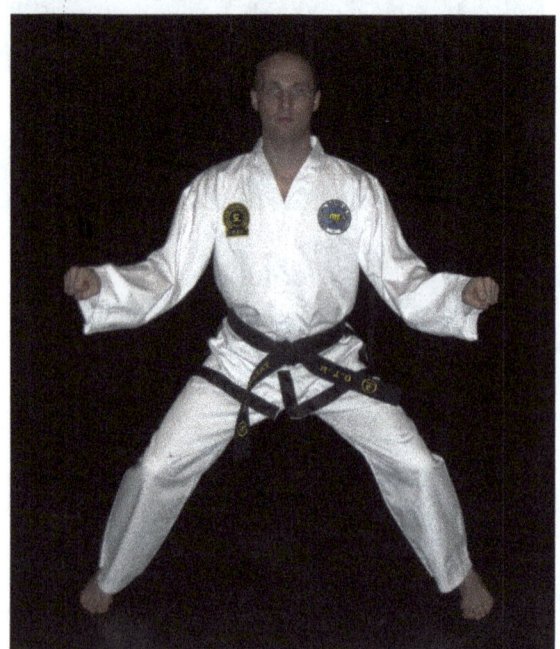

ANNUN SOGI
One and a half shoulder width

This stance is one and a half shoulder widths wide, both toes pointing forward.
Pay attention to these aspects:

1. The bodyweight is distributed over both legs.
2. The knees must be pressed outward; the kneecap must be in line with the ball of the foot.
3. Make sure the back is straight by making a sitting movement.

X-Stance *(Kyocha Sogi)*

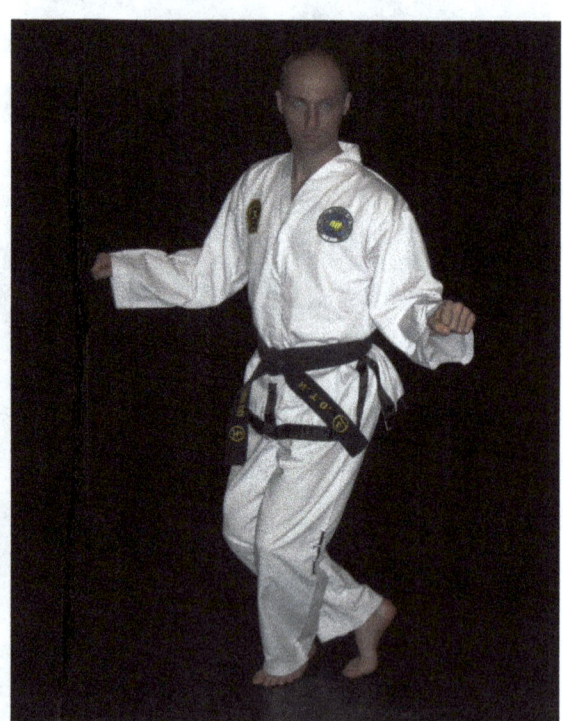

6. Practical Taekwon-Do

Rear Foot Stance (*Dwitbal Sogi*)

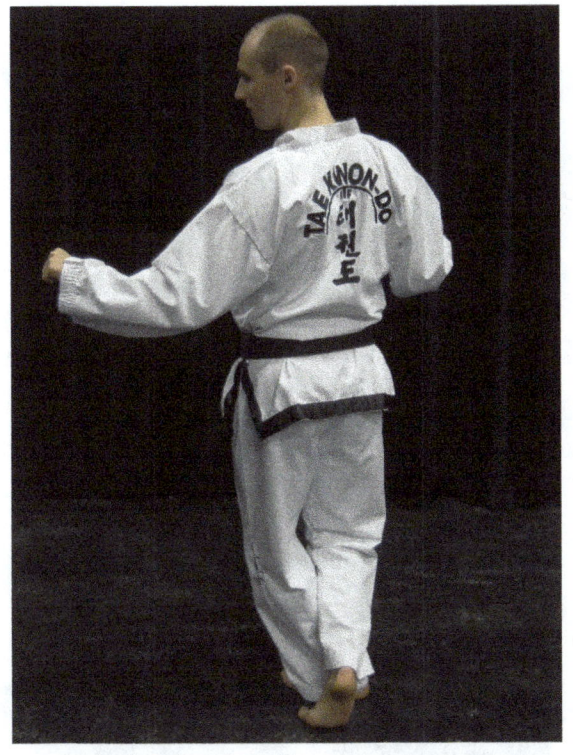

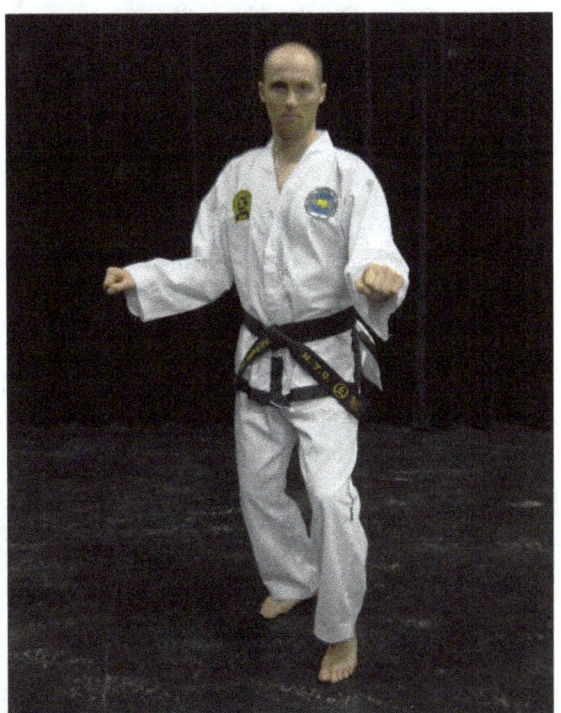

KYOCHA SOGI

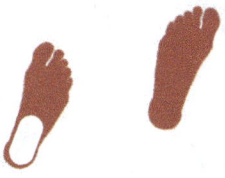

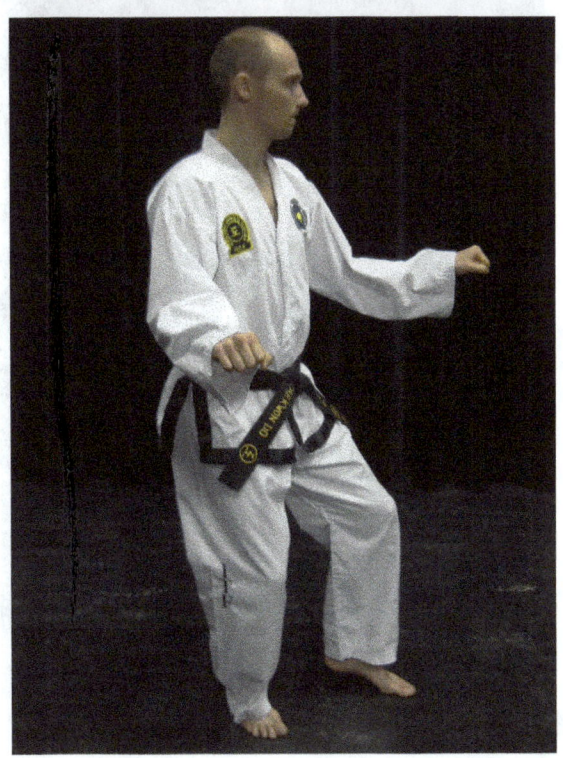

This stance is very effective if one wants to quickly change direction in the same place (turning around the longitudinal axis). One should pay attention to the following aspects:

1. 90% of the bodyweight is on one leg.
2. The other leg crosses over this leg, making the ball of the foot touch the floor.
3. Both legs are bent.

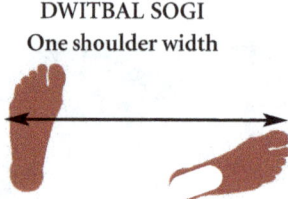

DWITBAL SOGI
One shoulder width

SOOJIK SOGI
One shoulder width

This stance is one shoulder width wide, both feet pointing slightly inward. Pay attention to the following aspects:

1. The rear leg is bent so that the kneecap is slightly over the toes.
2. The front leg is bent, the ball of the foot touches the floor.
3. 80% of the bodyweight is on the rear leg. This way, it is easy to perform a technique with the front leg.

Vertical Stance *(Soojik Sogi)*

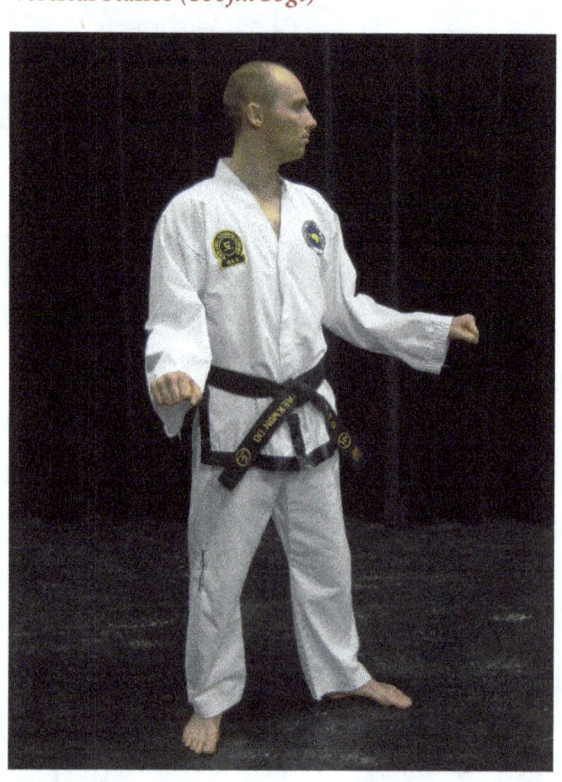

This stance is one shoulder width wide, both toes pointing slightly inward. Pay attention to these aspects:

1. The rear leg must carry 60% of the bodyweight, the front leg carries 40%.
2. Both legs are stretched to get as high as possible.

Bending Ready Stance *(Guburyo Junbi Sogi)*

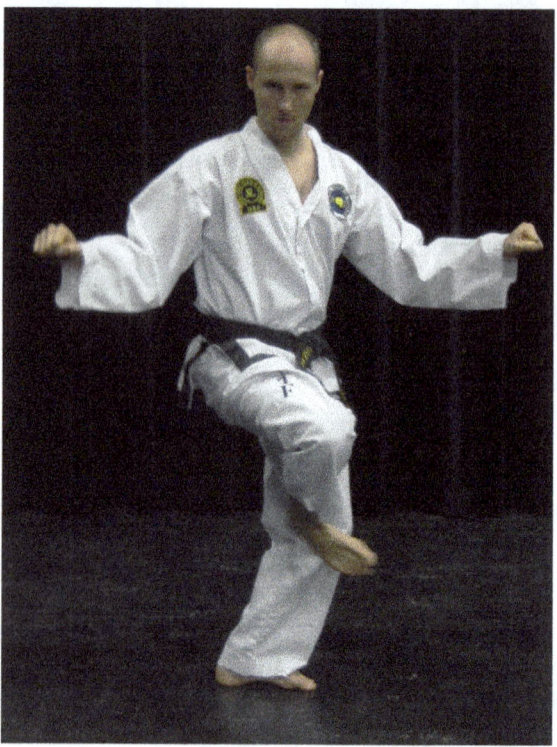

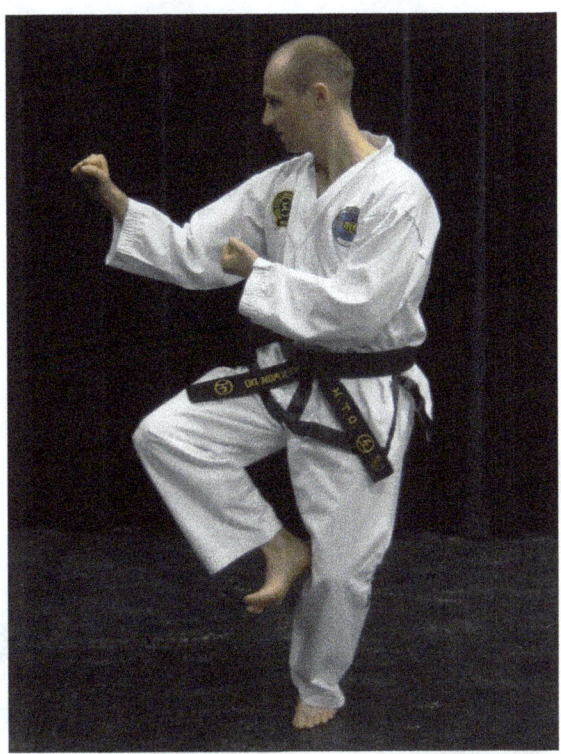

The bodyweight is on one leg, make sure the leg is slightly bent. The other leg is pulled up, the foot sole pointing toward the knee. The knee of the pulled up leg points slantingly forward. This stance is often used when making a side kick. The bending ready stance is performed explosively, and always in combination with a defensive block.

6.4 Starting points

Before a technique is executed, there is a starting point. By giving the attack or technique a starting point, one increases the impact on the eventual target. The starting point is the point from where the attack or block is commenced, but it is also the moment when the counter technique begins. In this paragraph, several starting points will be discussed.

Starting point with crossed arms

Because of the position of the arms, one creates maximum protection for the body from possible attacks. This starting point can be executed in two different ways:

Inside starting

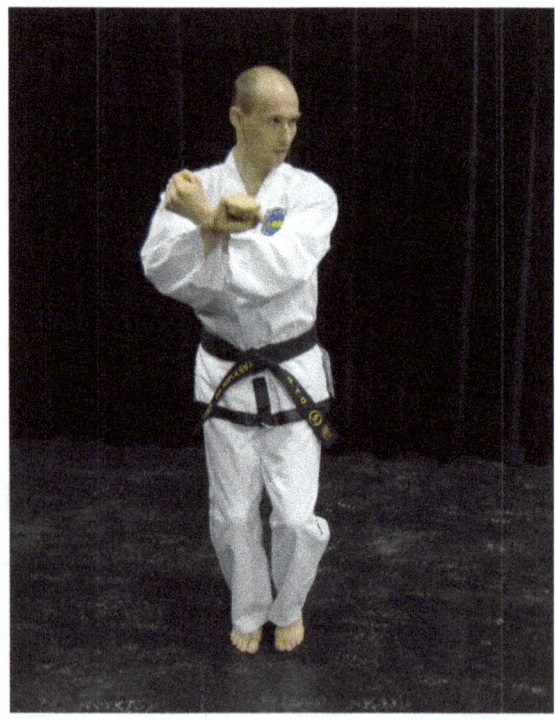
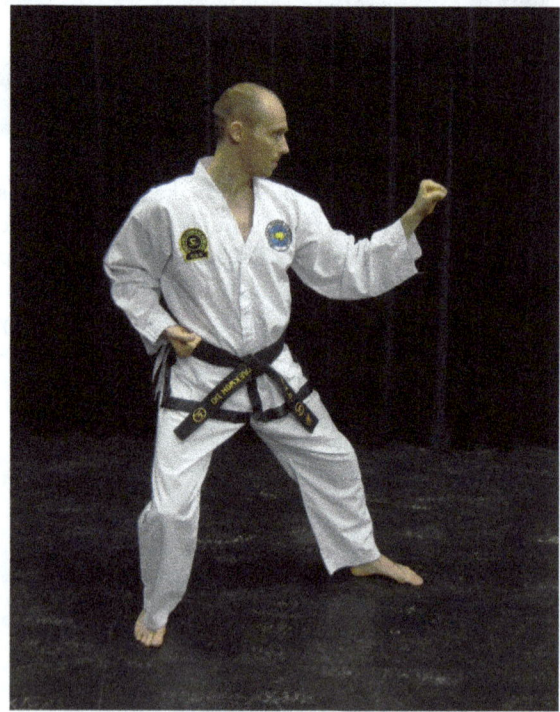

The attacking or defending arm is positioned between the body and the counter arm. When the attacking or defensive arm hits the target with the outside of the forearm or hand (the side of the little finger), then the starting point is on the inside.

Outside starting

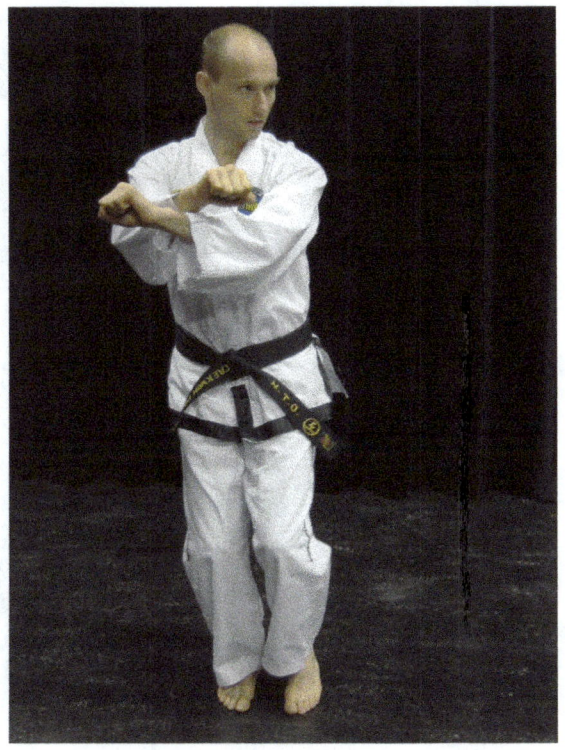 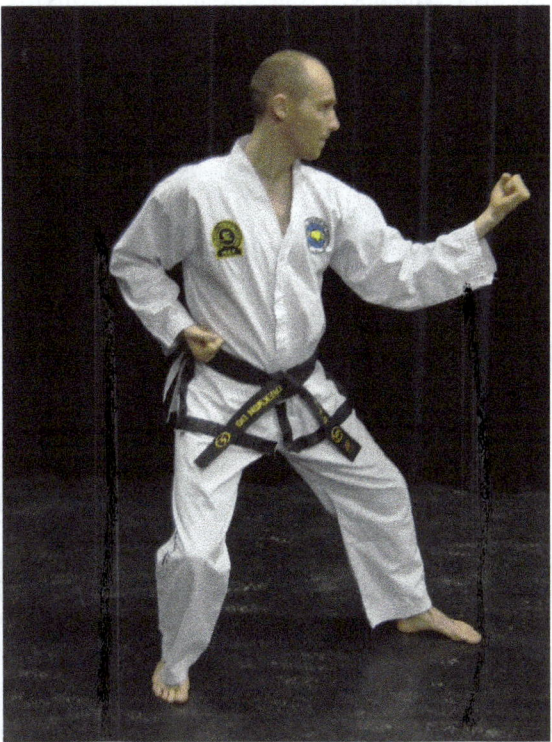

The attacking or defending arm is furthest away from the body.

When the attacking or defending arm hits the target with the inside of the forearm or hand (the side of the thumb), then the starting point is on the outside. This rule of thumb of inside and outside starting exists on behalf of a uniform execution.

Important points of interest during a starting point with crossed arms, with the body slightly twisted, are:
- Arms must be as relaxed as possible.
- The starting point is in front of the opposite chest (excluding some exceptions).
- Make sure the body is protected by the arms, so do not start too high.
- Make sure there is enough distance between the chest and the starting point; the starting point should not be too close to the body.

This causes the body to relax more and a greater motion can be reached, enabling for more strength development.

When the body is frontally positioned and one performs a technique, it is significant for the arms to be crossed in front of the chest, so that the distance to the target is equal on both sides.

Starting point

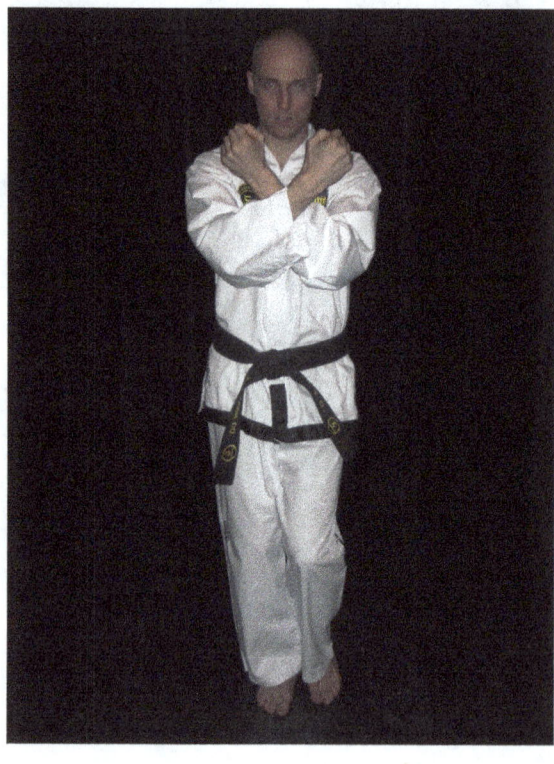

Ending point (wedging block)

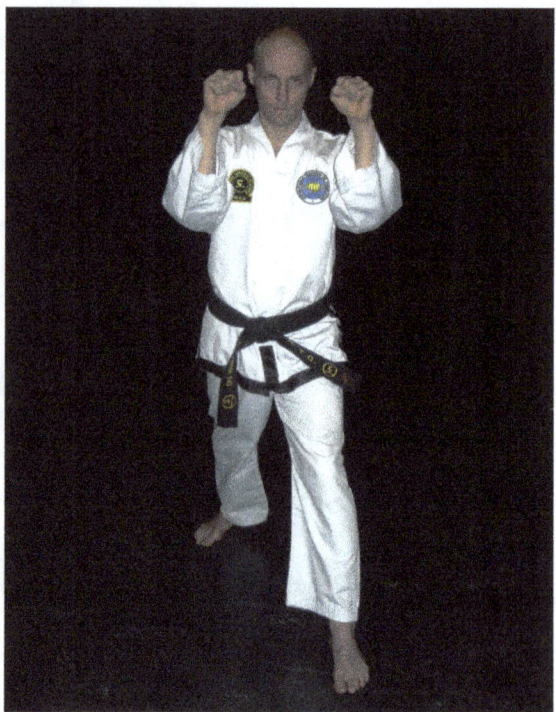

When one steps out with the left foot, during the starting point the left arm is closest to the body. The same principle applies to the right foot.

6. Practical Taekwon-Do

Starting point with both arms

This starting point is often used when performing double techniques such as a defensive block. This is a strong form of blocking because of the great motion.

Because the arm that does not block moves in the direction of the blocking arm, extra mass and force hit the target.

chest and the starting point; the starting point should not be too close to the body. This causes the body to relax more and a greater motion can be reached, enabling for more strength development.

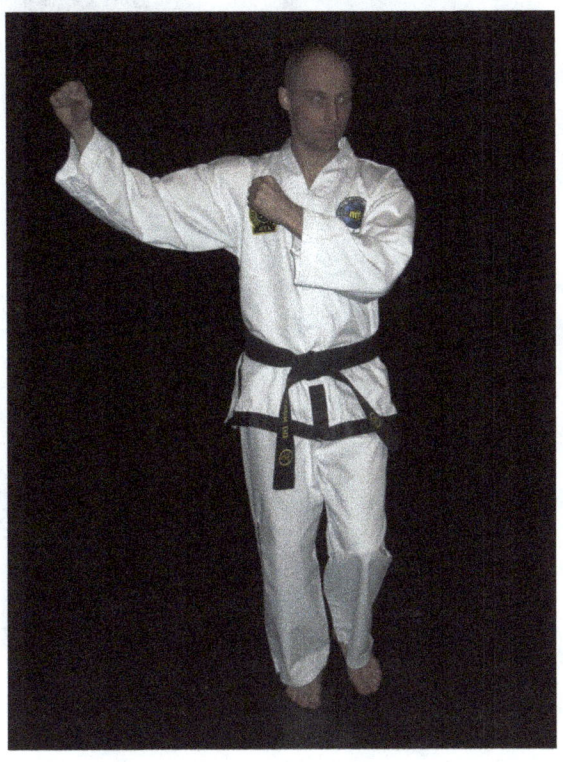

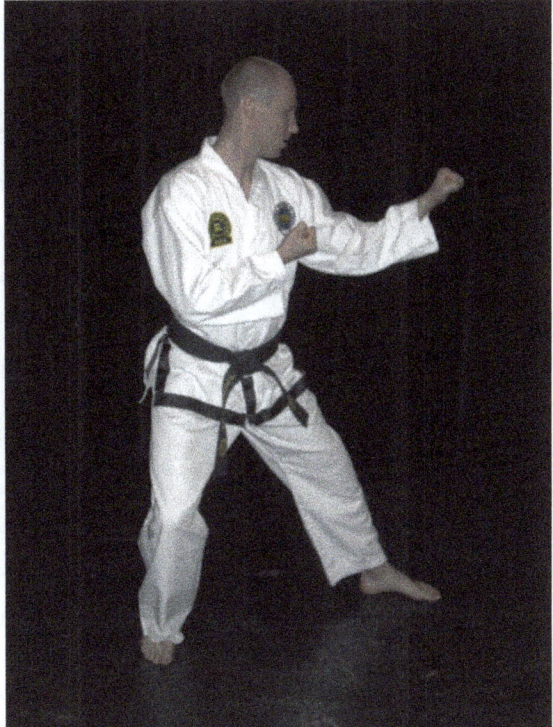

Defensive block

Look at the target during the starting point of the technique.

Important points of interest during a starting point with both arms, with the body slightly twisted, are:
- Arms must be as relaxed as possible. The starting point is in front of the opposite chest (excluding some exceptions).
- Make sure the body is protected by the arms, so do not start too far back or too far up.
- Make sure there is enough distance between the

Separate starting point

This starting point is often used when one is frontally positioned in relation to the opponent. One can think of a forward punch or an inward forearm block.

The left arm is pulled towards the hip. The right arm blocks.

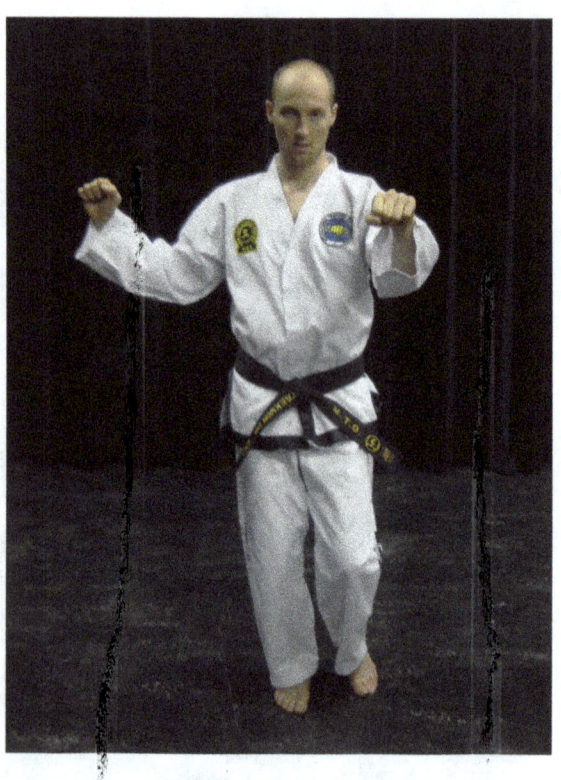

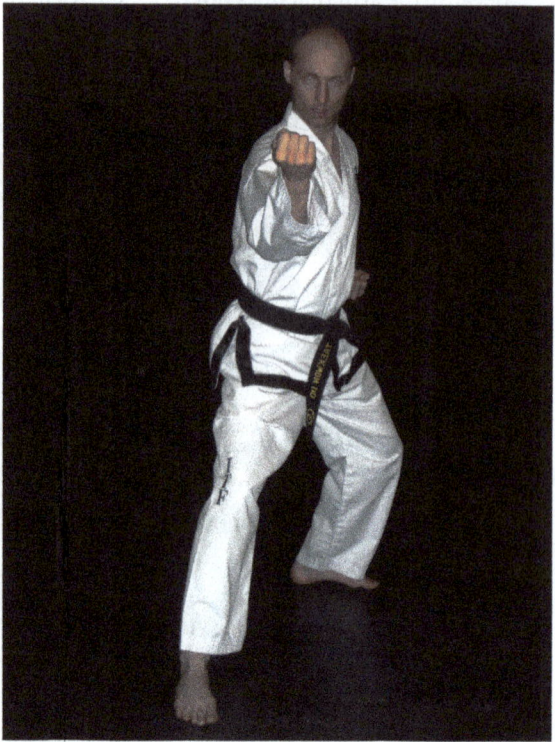

The left (counter) arm is relaxed and in front of the body. The right arm is at shoulder level.

An advantage of the separate starting point is that one uses the pectoralis major muscle and the pectoralis minor muscle (*Musculus pectoralis major and minor*). This is a very strong muscle group that can add much force to a motion.

Hip use

Muscles such as the leg, gluteal, and abdominal muscles are attached to the hip joint. It would be a shame not to make use of this, as all these muscles contribute to the development of mass, strength, and speed. The hip joint is the link between the upper and lower body. This is why a technique is not only performed with, for example, the fist; the whole body is used. Therefore, one should turn the hip in the direction from where the technique is made - there are some exceptions. There are many advantages in using the hip joint. One can use the hip upwards, downwards, and from left to right.

Turning movement

The turning movement is characteristic for many Taekwon-Do techniques. A turning movement in the technique creates a pure execution. It can be compared to the barrel of a gun; it has a certain structure that causes the bullet to come out twisted, which enables it to take its course as pure and stable as possible. Also, the turning movement creates acceleration; the technique hits the goal like a whiplash, which generates more force and gives the technique a penetrating effect.

Tightening and relaxing

Before one executes a technique, it is important for the body to be in a relaxed state. It is not until the moment that one hits the target that the relevant body part is tightened. Immediately afterwards one makes the body part return to a relaxed state. Too much tension on the body (the muscles) takes up strength and makes one slower; try to run when all the muscles of the leg are tightened. In a relaxed state, one is quicker and more agile.

Countermovement

According to Newton's law, every force has an equal and an opposite force. An example of this is that when one punches a wall with a certain amount of force, the wall 'gives back' the same amount of force. When an opponent walks into a side kick, he will receive the force of the kick, as well as the force he develops while stepping in. See also the subchapter 'reaction force' in the following paragraph. Furthermore, the countermovement creates balance in the exercise or technique.

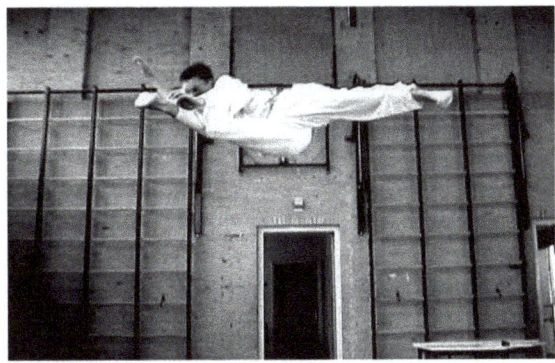

Twimyo Yop Bituro Chagi.

6.5 Strength development and starting points in Taekwon-Do movements

In this paragraph, two topics will be discussed more extensively. These topics are the theory behind the enormous and sometimes incredible force one can develop with Taekwon-Do techniques, and the basic principles that are applied to the different Taekwon-Do techniques.

Taekwon-Do distinguishes itself from many martial arts because it is a young martial art, based on science. Originally, martial arts were often passed on from father to son, which gave them a mysterious quality and emphasized the importance of tradition. However, the founder of Taekwon-Do has approached its development from a modern scientific perspective. Taekwon-Do techniques are based on kinetic energy; the energy of motion. The principles and laws of Isaac Newton have been incorporated in the development of Taekwon-Do, which has caused certain traditional techniques to undergo great developments concerning strength.

The following factors are themes concerning strength as developed by the founder. When a student understands and controls these factors, they are able to apply them to most Taekwon-Do techniques. There are other important elements in developing an optimal execution of a technique, which will be discussed later on in this paragraph.

Strength factors
- Reaction force;
- Concentration;
- Balance;
- Mass;
- Speed.

Reaction force
With 'reaction force' the authors mean retroactivity. As described before in the subchapter on starting points, every force has an equal and opposite force. If one throws a basketball against a wall with a certain amount of force, the wall returns this same amount of force to the ball.

During a fight, an 'innocent' punch can hit hard. If one makes a soft punch and the opponent is walking into the punch, the two forces are combined, which can make the punch very powerful after all. This basic rule is called reaction force.

Reaction forces are also present in a technique; the countermovement. If one uses a correct countermovement, it adds force to the technique. When one punches with the right fist, one should retract the left fist towards the belt. This creates more force.

Concentration
There are two elements that make up concentration:

Centralization
Centralization means that all forces are focused - or centralized - on one target, in order to achieve the greatest possible result. For example, when one executes a punch, all of the forces reach the vital part of the opponent through the knuckles of the index and middle finger. Or, for example; when one executes a side piercing kick, all forces are placed on the target through the outer edge of the heel. This is because the edge of the heel has a small surface and the heel has a firm bone structure. The following comparison illustrates this principle. If a heavy person stands on a glass sheet with large shoes, the sheet does not necessarily break. If a lightweight female stands on the sheet with stiletto heels, there is a greater chance that the sheet will break.

Joining
There are two ways of joining muscles in order to achieve maximum strength. One starts with the most important supporting muscles; the large muscle groups around the hip joint and abdomen. Before the technique begins, these muscles are tightened, and then the technique follows. The second moment of joining takes place at the moment of impact on the selected target. For this the smaller muscle groups are activated. Correct tightening and relaxing are very significant. One is not supposed to join all of the energy in the technique at the beginning of the motion.

Balance
As a martial artist, it is important to always be in balance. From this situation, one can react effectively in an attacking and defending manner. Balance is also significant for the maximization of techniques. In subchapter 6.3 (Stances), the importance of the right stance has already been discussed. When a stance is correct, one can not only react in an attacking or defending manner; consciously incorporating balance into the posture can make the difference between a technique that works and one that does not. The authors often see the execution of a side kick with the heel of the back foot being off the ground. This does not only increase the chance of falling or being tipped over; it also causes one to lose a lot of strength. This is also the case for a punch in walking stance where the heel of the back foot is off the ground. Much energy flows away through the heel, instead of being directed at the opponent. With a correct posture (stance), the reaction force from body to floor is the greatest. In both cases, the

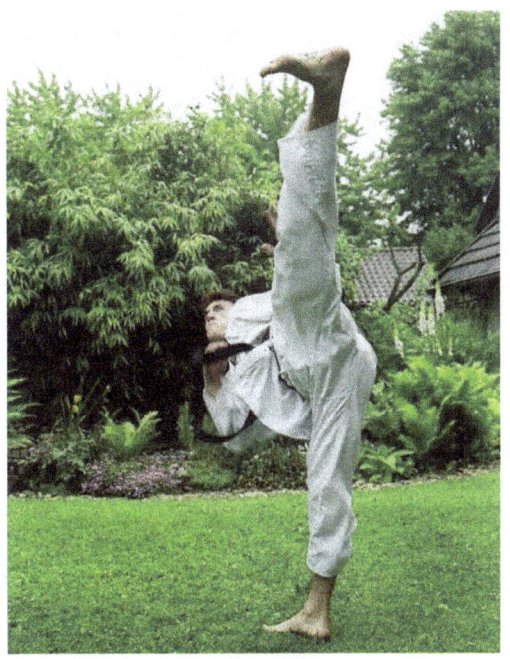

Nopunde Yopcha Jirugi.

heel needs to be firmly planted on the floor.

Mass

In this case, mass means bodyweight. In physics, the largest possible mass together with the factor speed causes movement energy or force. In the theory of motion, every weight becomes heavier when it is in a downward motion. This is caused by gravity (the attraction of the earth). Taekwon-Do uses this principle. When standing or in motion one often makes one's mass go downward, so that more mass and therefore movement energy can go into the technique. At the moment of impact, the center of gravity descends and the bodyweight 'falls' into the technique in a controlled manner. By using the hip in order to accelerate, one creates more mass. Through the muscles around the pelvis and the abdomen, the hip is turned in the direction of the attack or defense, which increases the bodyweight that is moving in the direction of the target.

Example: How to do this standing in a gunnun sogi (walking stance)?

The 2nd movement from Do-San (3rd tul) is used as an example. When standing in a walking stance, one slightly bends from the back knee joint, making the heel come off the ground so that the hip can easily turn inwards. Then, one brings the body up slightly and descends into the correct position. At the same time the punch is executed.

To make maximum use of mass, punches at or under one's own shoulder level are preferred. A side kick under one's own hip level is more powerful than abve one's hip level. This is why during a flying side kick it is important to 'gain height', so that one can kick under one's own hip level. Too frequently, people hang backwards or kick too high, which leaves little force for the movement. Oftentimes one simply does not jump high enough.

The damage a punch or kick can cause when using one's own mass is far greater than with a technique where one only uses an arm or a leg. After all, the damage a heavy bus can cause is much greater than the damage a car can cause (at the same speed).

Breathing

Breathing is essential for life. With a correct and controlled way of breathing, one can influence stamina. In sports, breathing is very important as well; power lifters and tennis players for example are often clearly heard and seen on television when they are breathing. Through a correct way of inhaling, a moment of relaxation is created. Relaxation - and through this mental and physical peace before a technique - is important. It enables one to correctly prepare a movement and to quickly and optimally execute it. A correct way of exhaling can add force to a technique. With a sharp exhale, one tightens all of the abdominal muscles, which means that more strength can be put into the technique. Also, one is able to endure more; the pain will be less if one is hit when the (abdominal) muscles are tightened, and the internal organs are better protected as well. This

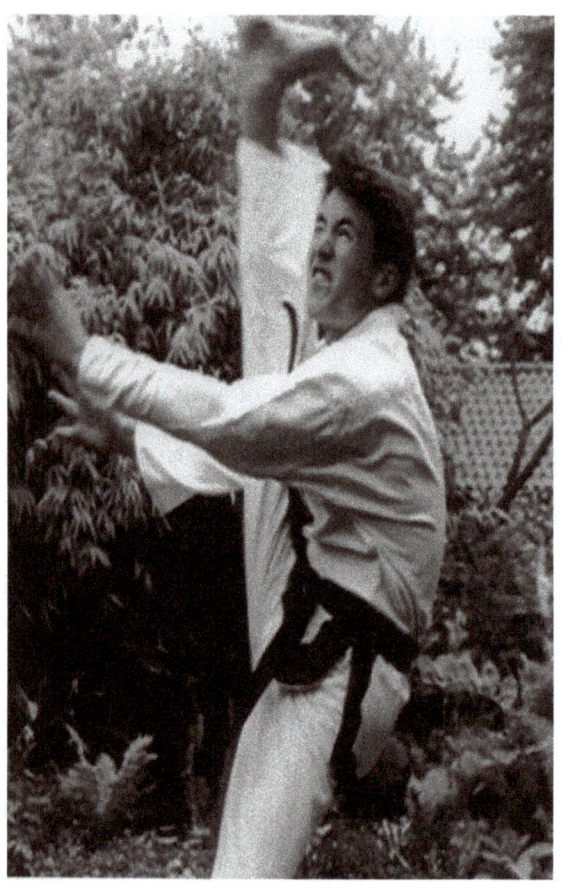

is why one sould never inhale at the moment of a block or attack.

Speed

Although all the aforementioned factors are important; the most important factor in strength development is speed of movement. Two principles will be discussed here: 'speed as effectiveness' and 'speed is force'.

1. Speed as effectiveness

In the 70s of the previous century, the founder has had research done on speed. This research has shown that a correct and fast Taekwon-Do attack cannot be blocked. This has to do with the speed of the attacking technique and the reflex speed of the opponent. The execution time of the attack is shorter than the time one needs for a reflex with a block that follows. It needs to be mentioned that it requires a lot of training to actually be able to execute the attack techniques this fast.

2. Speed is force

In the theory of motion, the force or energy of a movement is described in a formula:

$$\text{Force (energy)} = \text{mass} \times \text{speed}^2$$

Force is determined by the mass of the moving person multiplied by the square of the speed of the person. If a person kicks a break board with a certain speed and mass, it amounts to a certain force. If another person kicks the board with the same speed, but with twice the amount of mass, the force (or energy) of the kick will be twice as much. If one kicks with the same mass but with four times the speed, the force of the kick will be four times four as much force. This explains why a light Taekwon-Do student can develop an enormous amount of strength, as long as they are fast as lightning.

It speaks for itself why a slender, muscular arm is much quicker than a big, sturdy arm (an F16 plane can ascend quicker than a Boeing 747). Since it is easier to accelerate the end speed of the light arm, it is very useful to train moving speed instead of muscles!

There are several different types of speed that can be distinguished when executing the tuls:

Normal motion

This indicates a normal movement, which means that there is a normal tempo between two movements, with one breath. In this book, this is the movement that is meant when there is no specific mention about the execution. This is the primary form for the execution of all fundamental exercises. It is the only form a new student encounters, since it is the only form that the two preparatory tuls (*Saju Jirugi* and *Saju Makgi*) and *Chon-Ji* tul have.

Slow motion
Slow motion means a slowly executed movement. This movement also has a slow manner of breathing. There are no exact times, but the movement and breathing must be slower than normal. This puts an emphasis on a movement, because of balance, muscle control, control, or as a breathing exercise. The hand and foot movements end at the same time.

Fast motion
Fast motion means that the movements are quick. This concerns the time between two movements, which is shorter than usual. The manner of breathing remains normal. This mainly concerns two attack techniques, where there is inhaling and exhaling.

Continuous motion
This means a continuous or combined movement. There is no interval between the end of the first and the beginning of the second movement. During these movements, one inhales one time and exhales twice. Similar to the movements, the breathing continues and is equally divided between the two movements. This mainly concerns two defense techniques.

Connecting motion
This signifies a connected or joined movement. Similar to the continuous motion, there is no interval between the two movements. The movements cross over. Breathing, however, is different. With a connecting motion, one breathes in once, exhales about 30% during the first movement, and the remaining 70% during the second movement. This puts the emphasis on the second movement. It mainly concerns a defense technique that crosses over into an attack technique, where the first part is mostly flexible, and the second part is mostly quick

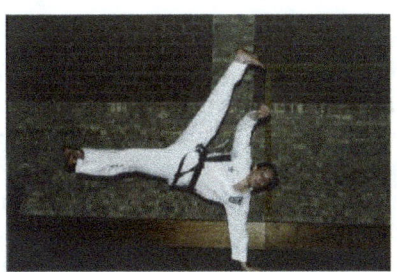

Additional elements
Apart from the aforementioned six elements, there are other elements that play a role in the successful execution of a technique. These elements will be discussed next. All these factors need to be executed rhythmically, coordinated, and flexible, and at the same time. Only then can it be called a complete movement. One can develop maximum strength through this 'complete movement'. It takes a lot of training, patience, and studying, before a Taekwon-Do student can truly understand and apply these factors.

- Interception and reactive power;
- Turning;
- Relaxation-tension (rhythm);
- Muscular tension;
- Snap movement;
- Sine wave motion;
- Flow;
- The art of thinking without thinking.

Interception and reactive power

Interception is very significant. The alert Taekwon-Do student may notice that in a lot of tuls, one steps in the direction of the opponent. When a punch or kick is intercepted by a block, hold, throw, or counterattack, it means the opponent was not able to optimally execute the technique. In other words, the movement momentum of the attack technique is off. It is probable that the opponent was surprised. Interception has to do with reactive power, which can very well be trained. In the theme 'speed as effectiveness' it has already been mentioned that the reaction speed is always slower than the execution time of an attack. This is why it is important to keep a close eye at the opponent at all times.

Turning

Many Taekwon-Do movements include turns. Turns create a pure and correct movement. See also 'Starting points' in subchapter 6.4. But a turn also causes acceleration. If one wants to break a board with a heel kick, one can rotate around the longitudinal axis to generate extra force, increasing the chance that the board will break. Before the turn, one starts turning the arms and shoulders, which is followed by a turn of the head, the torso, the arms, the stomach, the pelvis, and the leg. The other leg, which is kicking, is swinging around like a pebble on a rope. Thus, one winds up like a spring, then releases a great amount of force all at once (turning = centrifugal force = acceleration).

Relaxation-tension

Taekwon-Do movements must be executed rhythmically. This has briefly been mentioned in subchapter 6.4. When one movement is completely finished, the next one begins. This way, there is a continuous flow of energy, which consists of relaxation and tension. One can recognize the Taoist concept of yin yang, which is based on the assumption that the universe consists of a continuity of changes in energy.

Before the technique is executed, it is important that the body is in a relaxed state. The muscles do not tighten until the moment that the target is hit.

Muscular tension

As mentioned earlier, it is very significant that the muscles concerned are tightened at the moment that one hits the opponent. However, not only the muscles concerned are tightened; the entire body is tightened. This adds much force to a technique. Vice versa, one tightens the muscles at the moment of impact during an attack by an opponent. The muscles form a shield, decreasing the pain at the spot of impact and preventing (internal) injuries.

Snap movement

Many of the Taekwon-Do techniques include snap movements. This snap movement creates acceleration at the end of a movement. Because of this acceleration, the movement has a penetrating effect, which can sometimes cause internal damage to the opponent. Moreover, after impact the movement is retracted so quickly that there is very little chance for the opponent to grab on.

Many Taekwon-Do techniques can be executed in different ways. The side kick can, for example, be executed as a pushing, thrusting, pressing, or piercing kick. However, most of the time there is a combination of these which does not have the desired effect, making it easy for the opponent to grab the kicking leg. The traditional Taekwon-Do punch from the Chon-Ji tul (1st tul) is also executed differently in actual practice (not in the tul). The way the Chon-Ji tul describes the punch, it hits like a sledgehammer. However, this punch can also be executed with a snap movement (explosive execution and pulling back immediately after impact). This way, the punch can do more internal damage. This form of execution is preferred when the technique has to be applied during an actual fight. The opponent will not be able to grab the arm. In both cases, the fist needs to be turned inward at the very last moment.

Sine wave motion

The sine wave motion is used during the execution of many Taekwon-Do techniques. By means of the knee joint, one can relocate one's mass during a movement and increase one's speed, which eventually creates more force. One creates downward and upward motions; the so-called sine wave motions. The motion must be flowing, natural, and easy, which emphasizes the importance of relaxation and tension.

Flow

It is difficult to describe exactly what flow is. It refers to a state of mind, in which a person is completely absorbed by what they are doing. It is characterized by focused energy and activity, complete involvement, and perception of success. Hungarian-American psychologist Mihaly Csikszentmihalyi has done much research on this topic. Flow is important for athletes in general, but also for martial artists such as Taekwon-Do students. Someone who is *in a flow* could be described as 'completely immersed' or 'invincible'. In other words, one transcends oneself, and everything is *in place*.

Characteristics of flow according to Csikszentmihalyi:
- A clear goal;
- Concentration and singleness of purpose;
- Loss of self-consciousness: one is completely involved in the activity;
- Loss of sense of time;
- Balance between one's own skill and the activities that need to be done: the activities are not too difficult, but very challenging;
- A sense of personal control over the activity;
- The activity is intrinsically rewarding.

It is important to try to get in the flow, especially for Taekwon-Do students that engage in matches or students that have exams. When the mind is empty and focused, the body can be brought to the correct moment.

The art of thinking without thinking

Several stages of development can be identified in Taekwon-Do. One of the most important stages is when someone stops thinking and starts feeling. One thinks without thinking, as it were. All movements are quick and reflex-like. One feels what is happening and responds accurately. This stage is not necessarily synchronized with the achievement of the black belt; it takes years of training and study. In the authors' opinion, it is significant for a martial artist - in this case a Taekwon-Do student - to train the entire body and mind. This includes the mental aspect, the conditional-physical aspect, but also the numerous techniques.

6.6 Sparring

The authors consider it to be very important that a Taekwon-Do student is experienced in sparring. After all, Taekwon-Do is an art of self-defense. Sparring means the application of fundamental techniques in a (free) fight. It gives a good representation of one's learning developments, physical condition, insight, which techniques are used, if one is ready to fight, etc.

Sparring is a fight that is fought with adapted rules, in a standardized and controlled environment (see Figure 6.1), that is quite realistic – especially when one is 'fighting' an unknown opponent. During a Taekwon-Do match there are certain rules, of which the basic ones are listed below. For the complete match, coaching, and referee regulations the authors would like to refer you to the Referee Committee of the ITF Royal Dutch.

Illegal targets for attacks:
1. Back of the head (only hand techniques);
2. Neck, throat, throttle;
3. Armpits;
4. Back;
5. Below the belt.

Legal techniques:
1. All foot techniques;

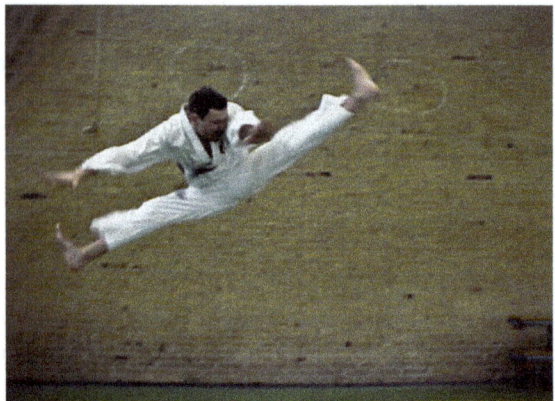

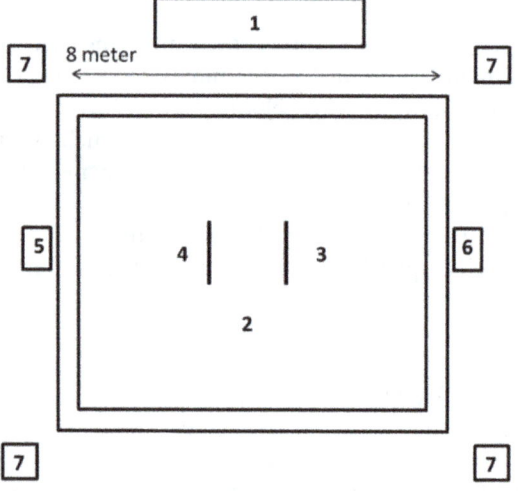

2. Front fist punch;
3. Back fist punch;
4. Reverse knife hand strike.

All other techniques are not allowed.

Scoring points
In order to score points, the following conditions must be met:
1. The used technique must be allowed;
2. On a legal target;
3. With enough force, balance and pulling back the applied technique;
4. With both feet starting and ending in the area designated for the match;
5. Between the start and stop signal made by the referee.

Score
For a correctly applied, legal technique, on a legal target, the score is as follows:

1 point for a hand technique on the body or head;
2 points for a foot technique on the body;
3 points for a foot technique on the head.

1. Table of general referee
2. Field referee
3. Blue Contestant
4. Red Contestant
5. Coach Red Contestant
6. Coach Blue Contestant
7. Corner referee

Figure 6.1 Competition field

Warnings
Warnings are given for:
1. attacking an illegal target;
2. using an illegal technique;
3. holding or restraining the opponent;
4. avoiding the fight;
5. turning one's back on the opponent;
6. having both feet outside of the match area;
7. simulating pain;
8. pushing with hands, shoulders, or body;
9. loss of balance (touching the floor with any part of the body but the feet);
10. uncontrolled way of fighting;
11. stalling;
12. pretending as if one scored by raising an arm;
13. touching the fist of the opponent before the sparring match has started;
14. talking to the opponent or the referee.

In case of an extension all warnings are cancelled.

Point deduction
Points are deducted for:
1. hitting an illegal target;
2. hitting a target with an illegal technique;
3. hitting too hard;
4. attacking an opponent while they are on the floor;
5. attacking before or after the referee's command to stop;
6. unsportsmanlike behavior toward the opponent, coaches and/or officials;
7. throwing the opponent;
8. not following the directions of the referee;
9. every third warning to the same person;
10. after three points deducted directly, the match is lost.

Unforeseen
When there is a situation that has not been classified for a warning or point deduction, the head or mat referee must assign a punishment that suits the offense.

Deciding a match with a tied score
When a match ends without a winner and it has to be decided, the following procedure takes place until the winner is decided:
1. an extension of one minute;
2. a second extension without a time limit, where the first one that scores points is the winner.

ALL GIVEN WARNINGS ARE CANCELLED IN CASE OF A PROLONGATION.

Several match definitions have been included in Appendix 1.

During a match, it is important to be right outside the fighting range of the opponent. This way, the opponent will have to cross a distance in order to attack, which creates enough time to react.

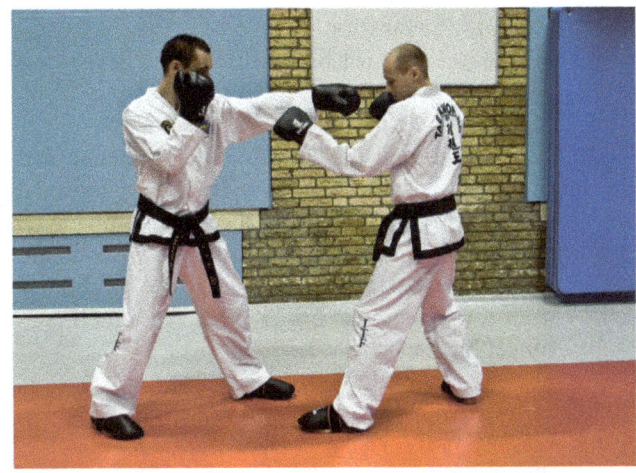

Above: Outside punching range
When one is within fighting range of the opponent, it is necessary to do something: block, attack, or avoid.

Below: Within punching range
The chance of hitting the opponent can be increased by a number of 'strategies'.

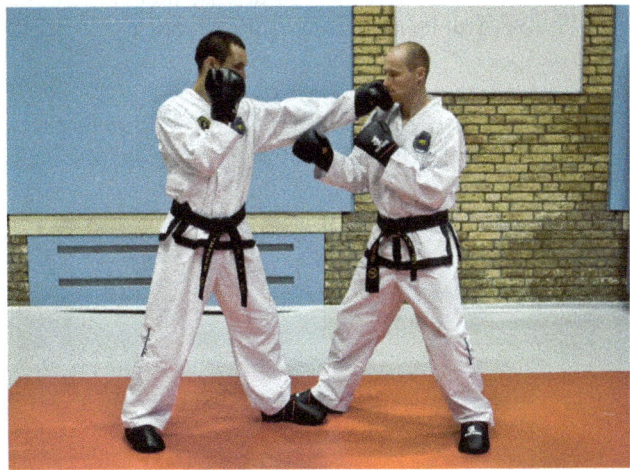

- Interrupting the opponent's attack;
- Applying a counterattack during the attack of the opponent;
- Counterattack;
- Making combinations;
- Making feints;
- Applying pressure.

These strategies will be briefly clarified next.

Interrupting the opponent's attack
Try to interrupt the attack of the opponent at the moment they are about to start. The big advantage is that the opponent will not expect anything to take place; the opponent has a strategy which is interrupted that beats them to the attack. With this technique, the opponent has to either cease their attack or get hit.

Counterattacking during the attack of the opponent
Since the opponent is busy attacking, their attention for defense will be decreased. Also, there is a chance that 'holes' will appear in their cover. Courage and using the correct technique are significant in this situation.

Counterattack
After the opponent has executed the attack, they will have to go back into defense mode. Since the opponent is busy returning to defense mode, there is an opportunity to execute a counterattack.

Making combinations
Through the use of combinations of different techniques, the chance of hitting the opponent increases. Since the opponent has to respond to the technique, holes will open up in their defense.

Making feints
By faking a movement a lot of information can be gained; what is the reaction of the opponent, where is their cover, how does the opponent move, etc. If an attack is aimed low, generally the opponent's cover will be low as well. The same goes for techniques that are aimed high.

Applying pressure
By applying pressure, the opponent will not have the opportunity to get in their rhythm, which makes their attack unconvinced and will create a mental advantage. Make sure to remain focused while applying constant pressure, as an advantage does not equal a victory.

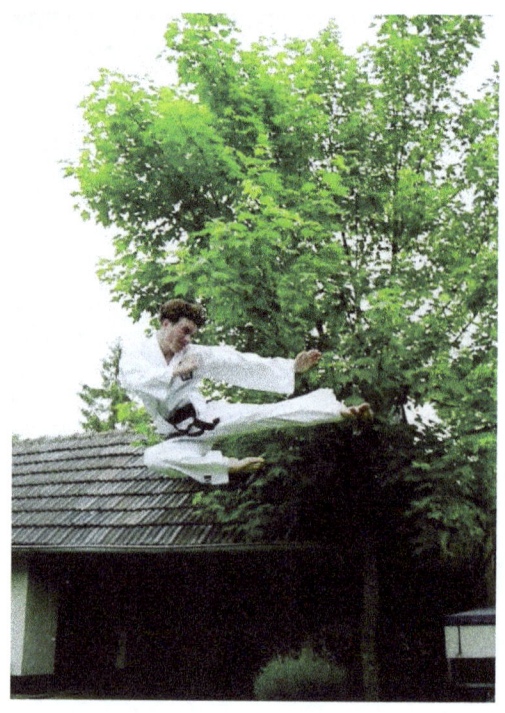

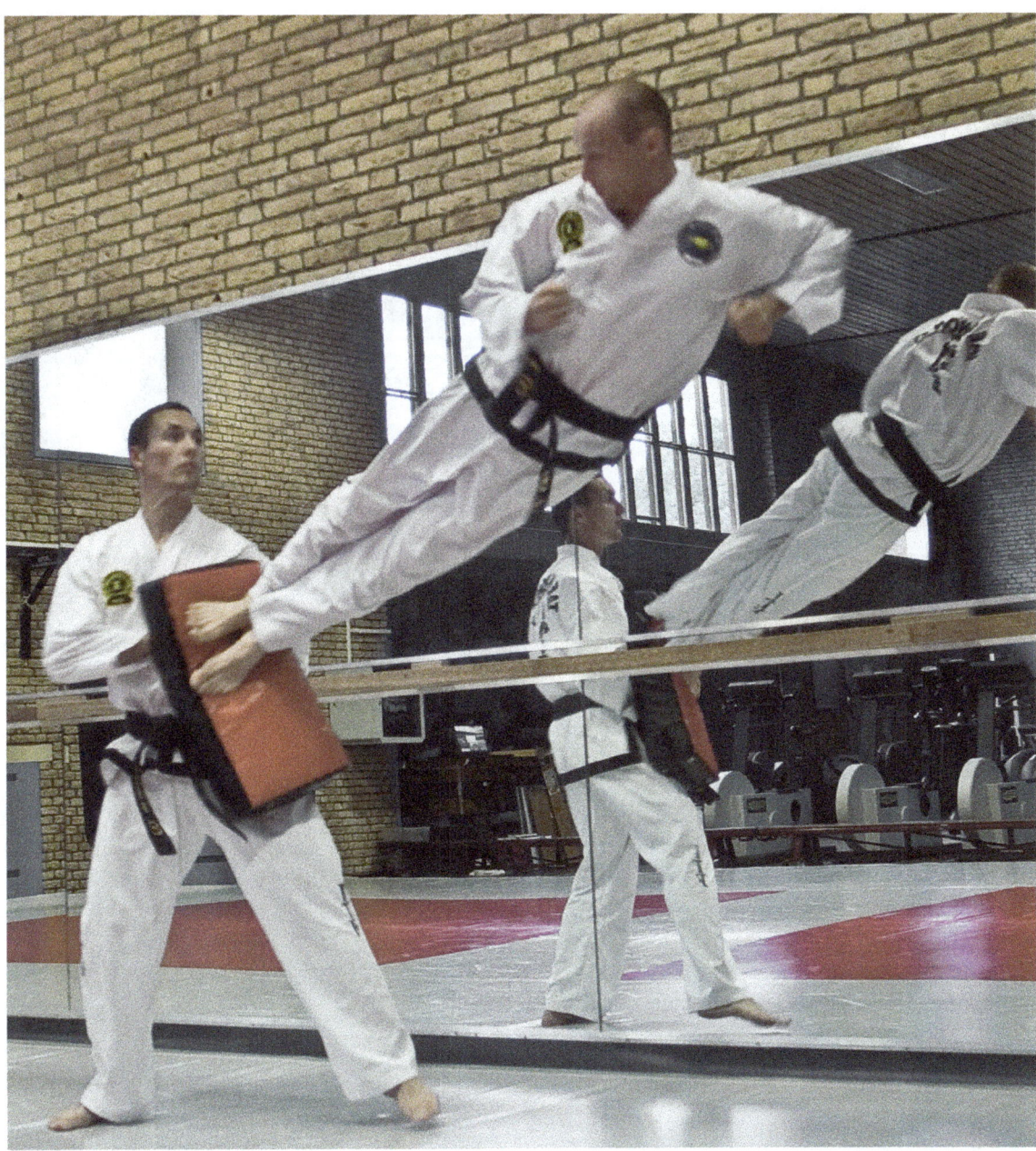

6.7 Flying techniques

Apart from the basic foot techniques, there are techniques that have a higher level of difficulty; flying techniques for example. Taekwon-Do is known for these (flying) leg techniques, but oftentimes not much attention is paid to flying techniques during Taekwon-Do lessons. The reason for this is that they are quite difficult and take up a lot of energy. Also, a correct execution by the instructor and a good

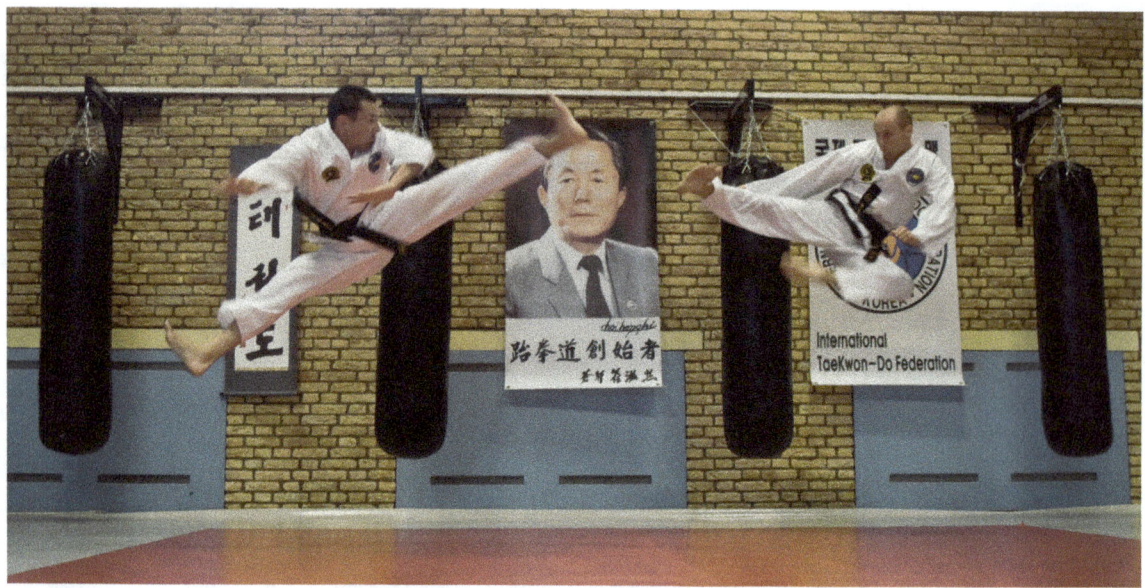

methodical composition during class are essential. The first goal is perception of success, and as with all techniques, one can only attain this by practicing very much. At a certain point, the techniques will start to feel good and comfortable, and they will provide a feeling of satisfaction – flying kicks included.

Possible reasons for using a flying leg technique are:
- attacking the opponent's body high and forcefully;
- crossing a distance;
- jumping over something.

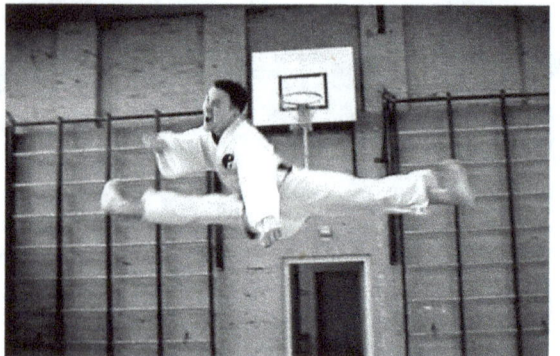

A flying kick can be very forceful, especially because it:
- uses gravity, since the kick is executed when descending;
- makes maximum use of the bodyweight;
- develops maximum starting power (in the jump);
- makes maximum use of turning speed.

Aside from these aspects, flying kicks also develop skills such as timing, balance, technique, awareness, and muscle strength.

Tips
Several tips for improving the flying kick:

HEIGHT
By actively raising the upward swinging leg, height is created. Swinging the arms upward also creates height; this technique is used in sports such as long jump, high jump, and basketball. Make sure not to aim the arms too high since this might negatively affect your cover. Aside from using arms and legs, it is important to slightly bend the knees before the jump is executed. This decreases the angle the muscle works under, so that more strength development

can take place. In a high jump for example, there is a take-off run in order to convert forward speed into height. For a Taekwon-Do student it is important to know that in order to create height, the take-off run should not be too long.

TURNING SPEED
By actively tilting the upward swinging leg (into the direction in which the rotation will be) one creates more turning speed. This is also applicable to the arms. Again, watch your cover. Using the hip is important with some flying techniques. Because of the sudden tilt in the body, the speed is increased.

After much training, one will notice that the jump consists of several phases:

- The starting phase, where one pushes oneself off;
- The ascending phase, where the body is lifted;
- The floating phase, also known as the dead center, during which one 'hangs' in the air for a brief moment;
- The descending phase, bringing down the body (because of gravity);
- The landing phase, where the body returns to its starting position.

By knowing which phase the body is in, it is easier to 'plan' the technique, which creates the opportunity to get even more from the flying kick.

Special techniques
If one wants to gain even more from the flying kick, one should add an extra turn, or perform more than one technique in the air. These techniques can be very spectacular. For example, one can make use of surrounding objects. It is important to slowly build up these techniques in order to prevent injuries. Several techniques are explained hereafter.

Twimyo 540 degrees Dollyo Chagi

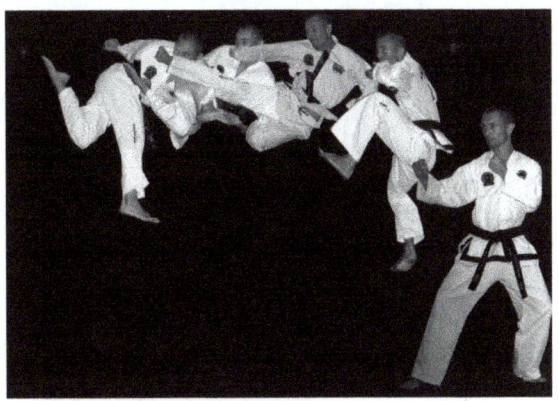

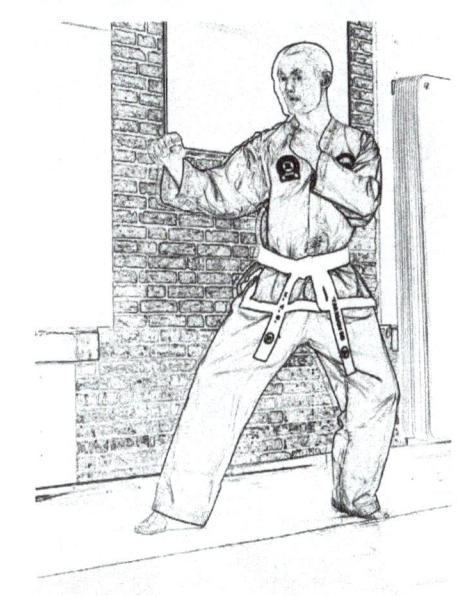

1. From this position, make a left turn of 180 degrees around the vertical axis.

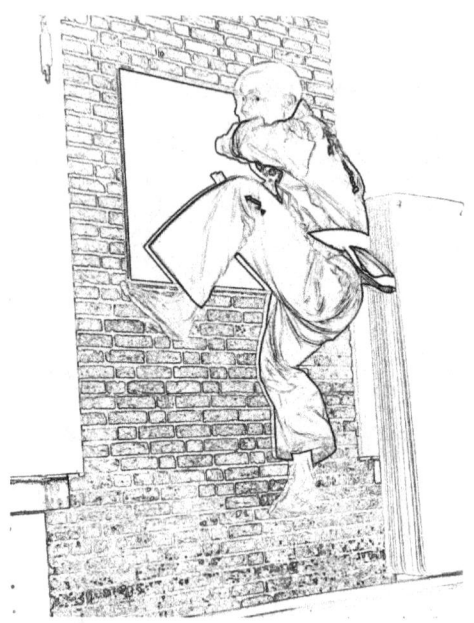
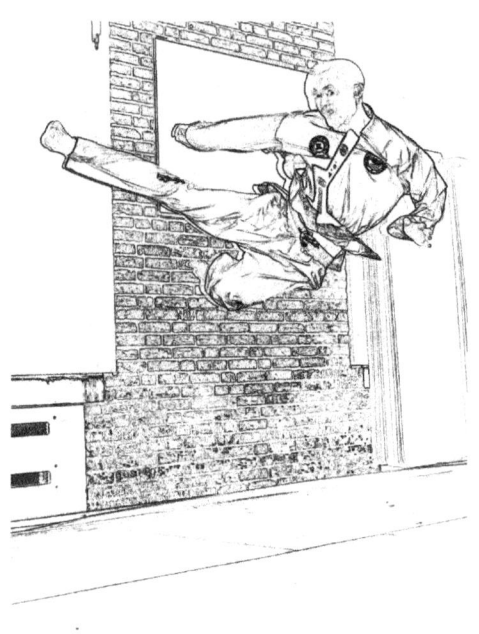

2. Lift the left knee (to increase height and extra turning speed).

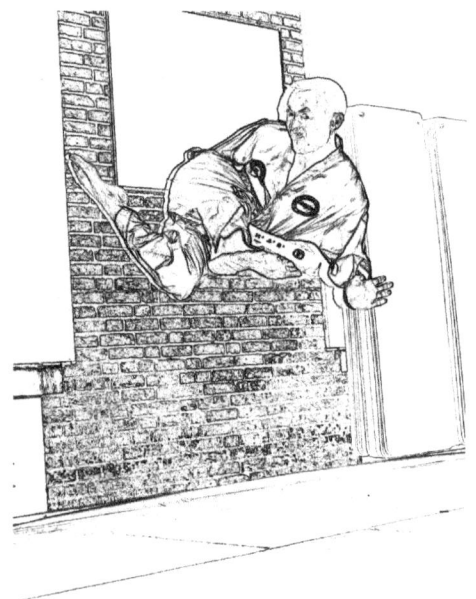
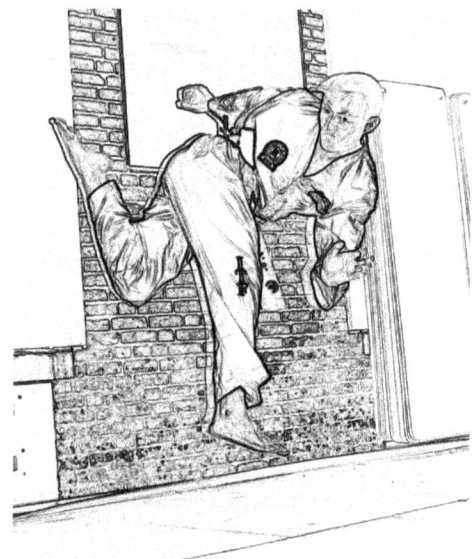

3. Make a turning kick with the right leg.

4. Land on the right leg.

Note: The attacking leg is the one that makes the kick and also the leg one lands on. Make sure the hip is used quickly at number 3.

Twimyo 540 degrees Bandea Dollyo Goro Chagi

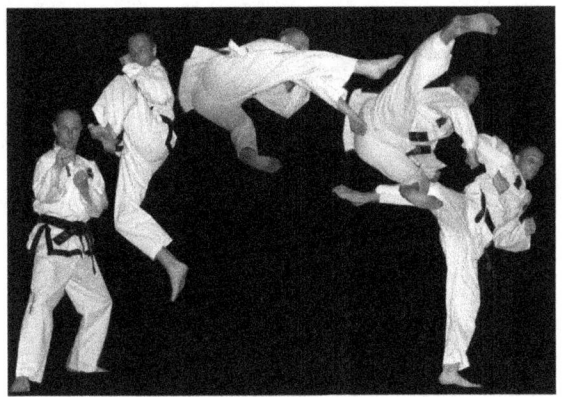

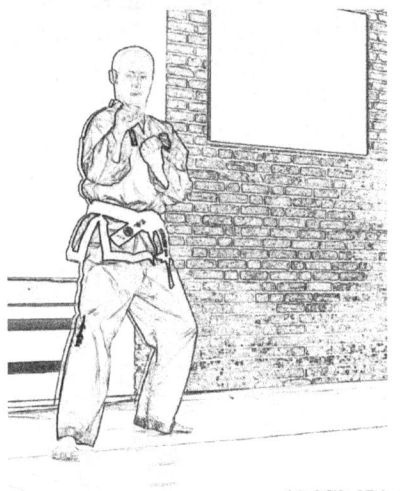

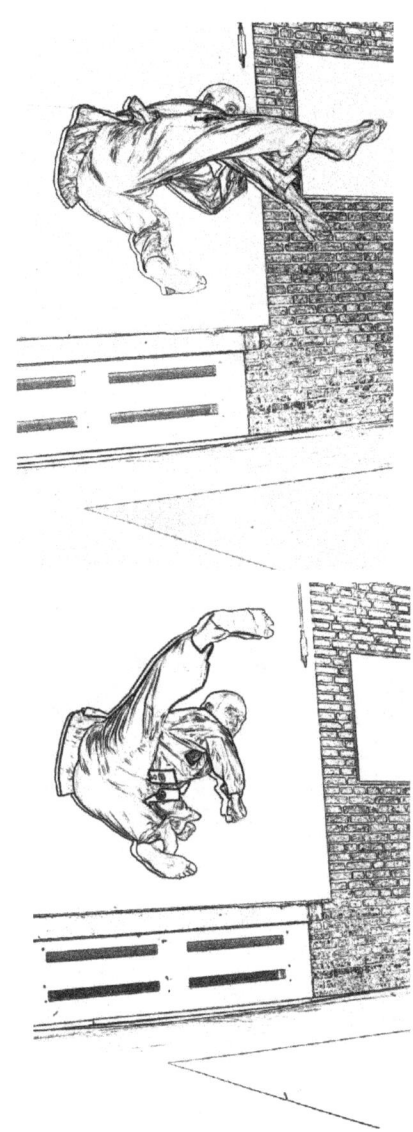

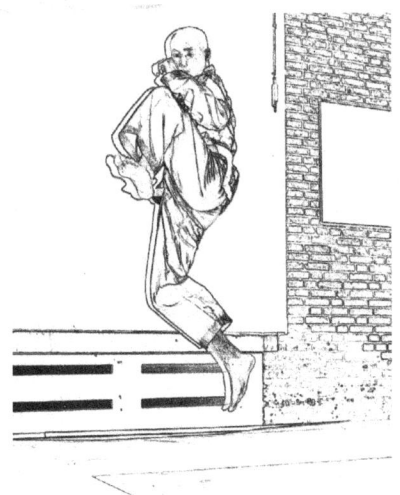

1. Lift the left knee upward in a slightly tilted manner (to increase height and turning speed).
2. Make a reverse hooking kick with the right leg.

Note: Shortly after lifting the left knee, the right leg is lifted off the floor.

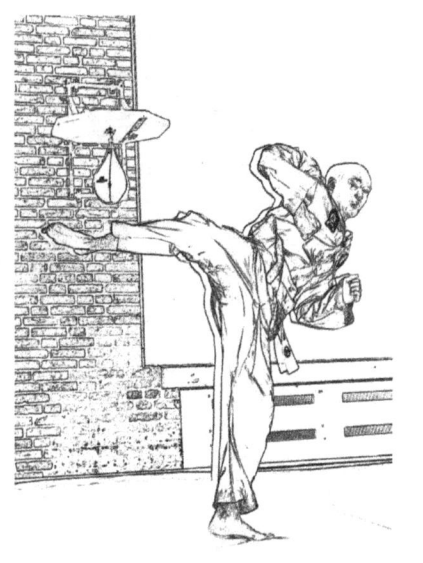

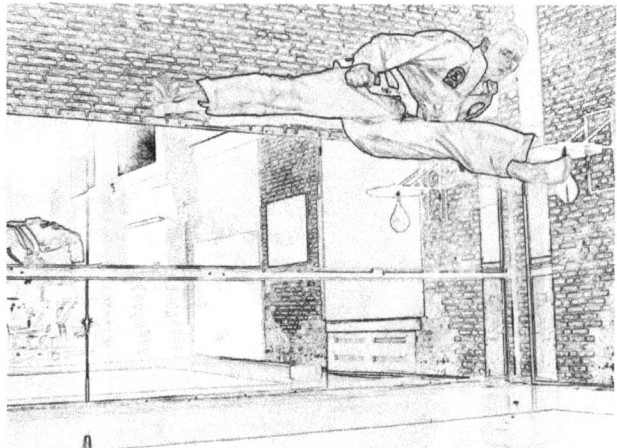

2. At the highest point of the jump, perform a twisting kick with the left leg, and simultaneously perform a side kick with the right leg.
3. After the kick, pull back the left and the lower part of the right leg.

Twimyo Yop Bituro Chagi (split kick)/Dollyo Chagi

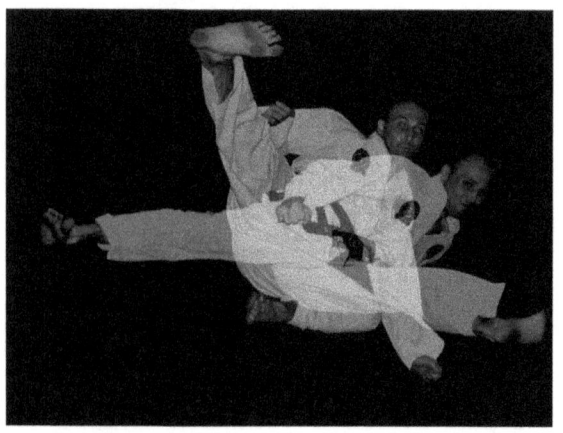

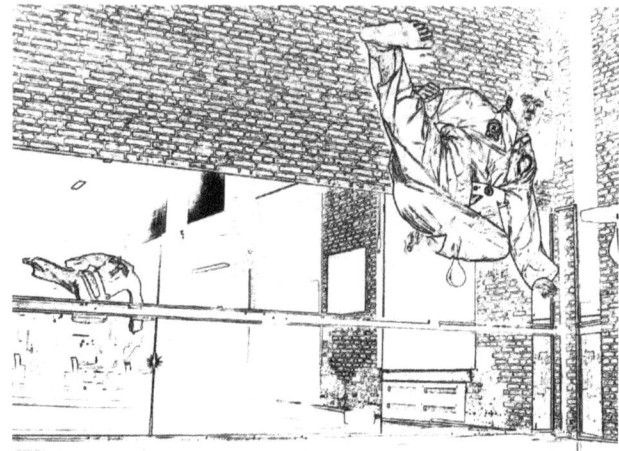

1. Use the left foot to push off and raise the right knee (to gain height).

4. Perform a turning kick with the right leg.

6. Practical Taekwon-Do

Twimyo I-Jung Dollyo Chagi

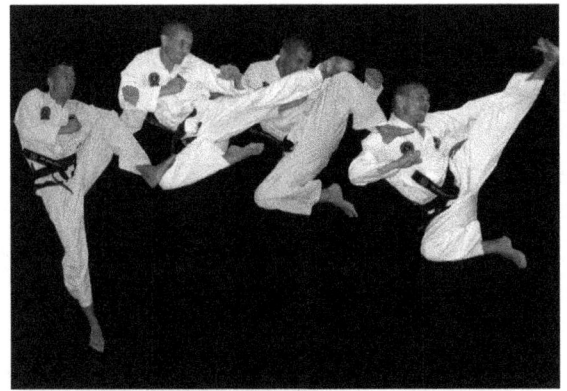

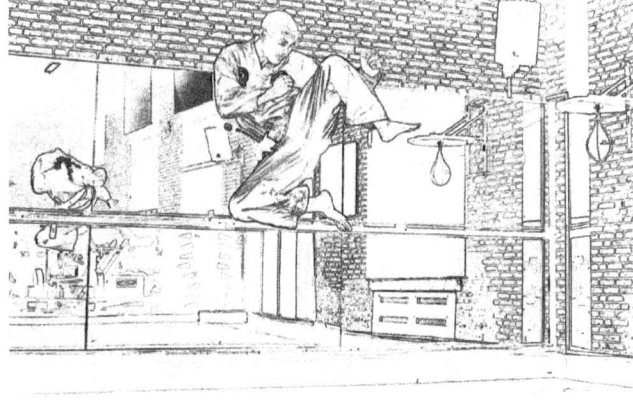

3. Quickly pull back the lower part of the left leg.

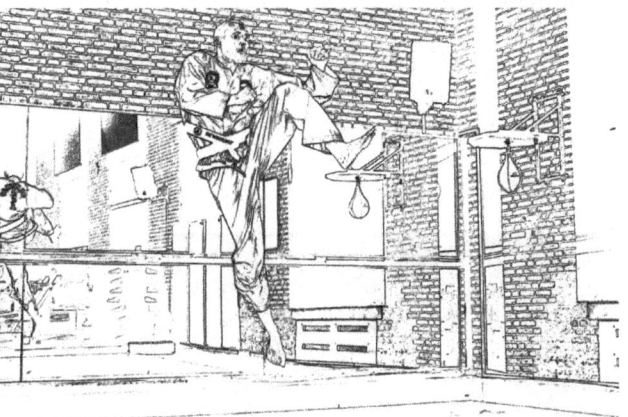

1. Push off with the right leg and lift the left knee.

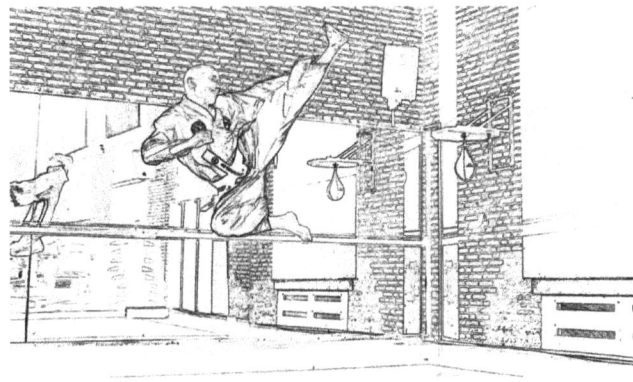

4. Perform another turning kick with the left leg.

Note: When executing a flying turning kick with the right leg, slightly move the right arm in the opposite direction. This helps to maintain balance and makes the kick more forceful.

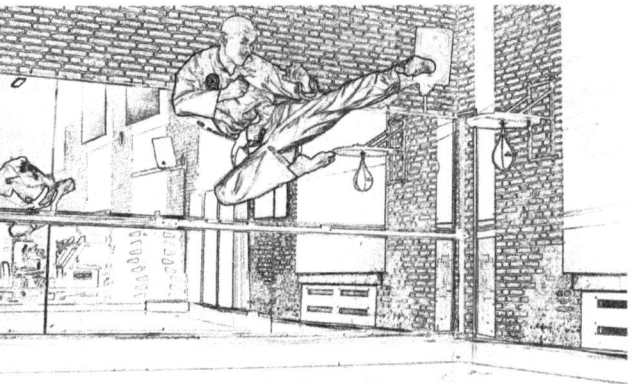

2. At the highest point, perform a turning kick with the left leg.

Twimyo Rasonsik Chagi (flying spiral kick)

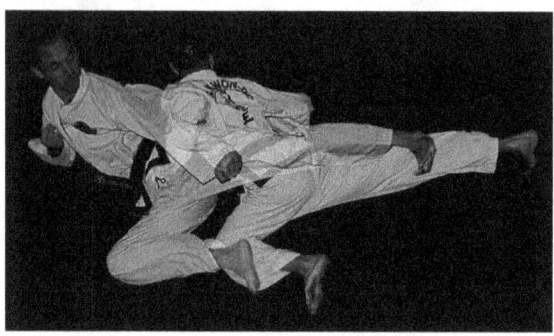

1. Push off with the right leg and lift the left knee.

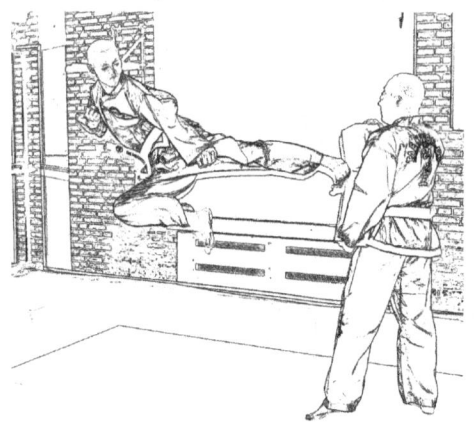

2. Perform a flying side kick with the left leg.
3. After the moment of impact, actively turn the hip and torso to the right

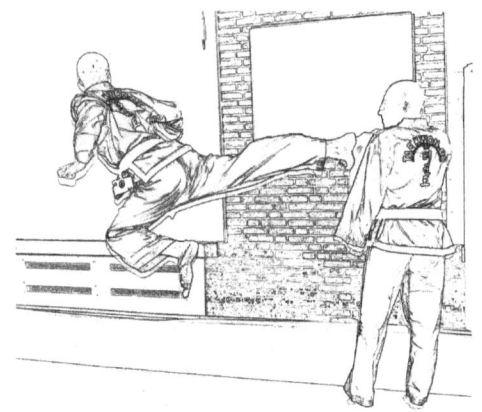

4. Pull back the left leg and perform a reverse kick with the right leg.

Note: It is important to rapidly turn the hip and torso while performing this technique.

Bansa Chagi (reflex kick: turning kick, using the wall)

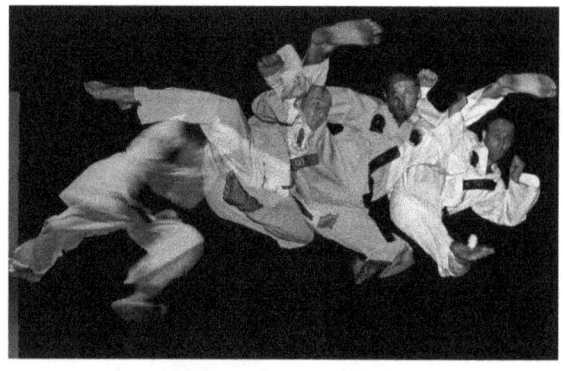

1. Make a short run and jump, using the left leg.

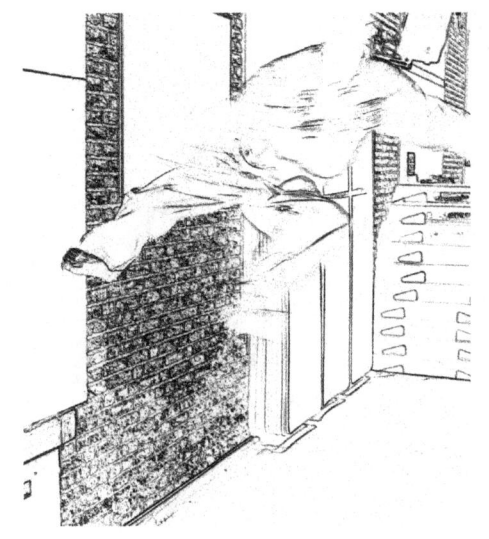

2. Place the right foot against the wall and use it to push off.

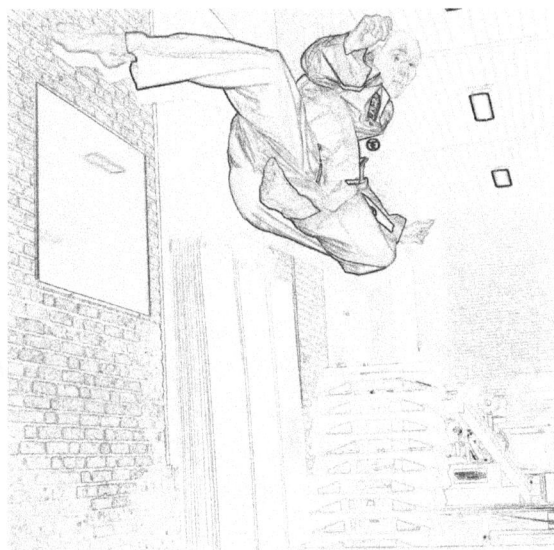

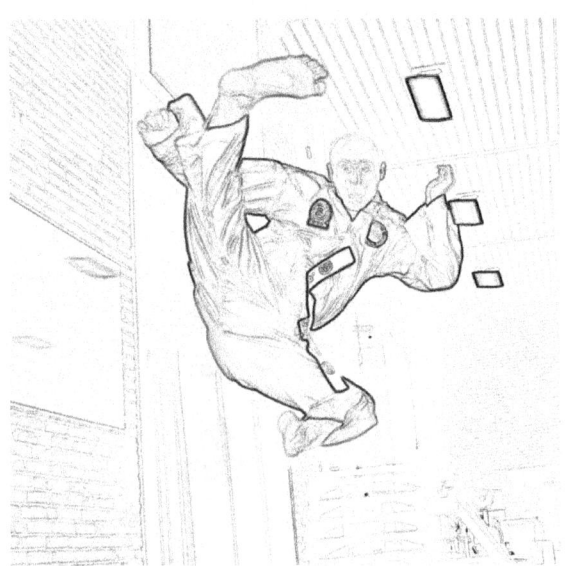

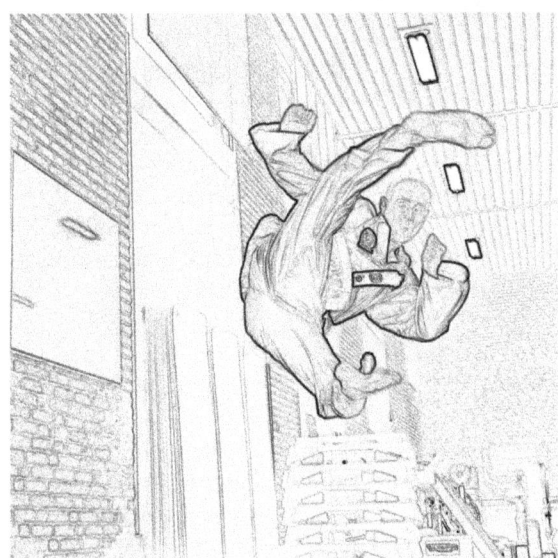

3. After this, perform a turning kick.

Note: Make sure that the run towards the wall is diagonal. Do not place the right foot too high on the wall. This way, there is an opportunity to create more height, providing one with more time to perform the kick.

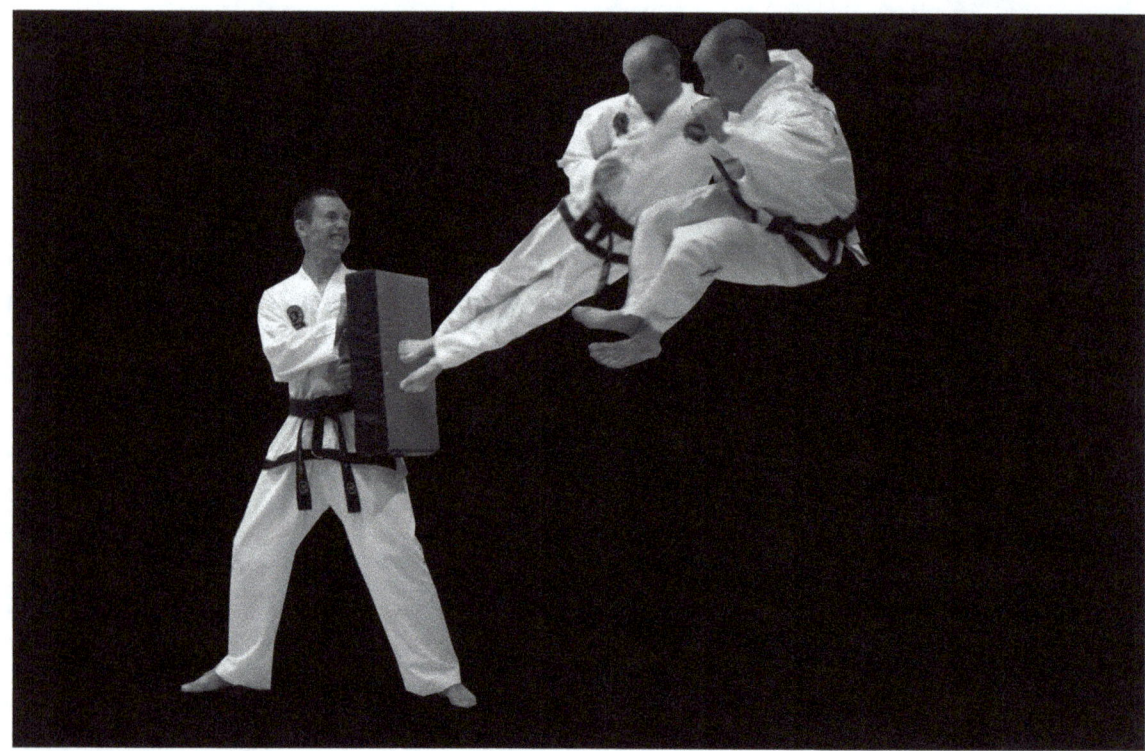

Apart from a wall, one can push oneself off of a person or another object. Furthermore, instead of a Dollyo Chagi other kicks can be used as well. The notion behind this technique is to be able to quickly change attack direction via an object.

6.8 Break tests up to the 1st dan

The speed, strength, precision, and effectiveness of several Taekwon-Do techniques is tested by means of a break test. Break tests can be performed on several different materials, such as wood, roof tiles, glass, or stone. Glass, roof tiles, and stone are often used during demonstrations because of the impressive effect they have. Wood is often used during a demonstration in order to demonstrate difficult techniques. In general, break tests are divided into two categories:
- Power break tests;
- Precision and control break tests.

Power break tests

The goal of a power break test is to break as many objects as possible, or an object that is as hard as possible. Oftentimes the entire body mass is used for this. During these tests, the point of application of the force barely moves. In other words, the place where the force of the technique focuses on stays the same, which maximizes the effect of the force. If one is holding one or more plastic boards, one needs to ensure 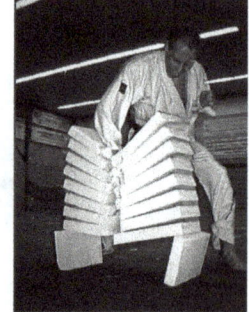 that the board does not yield. Examples of power breaking are breaking as many concrete bricks as possible, or to break as many plastic boards as possible in a break test holder. The force and impact of a technique are tested specifically.

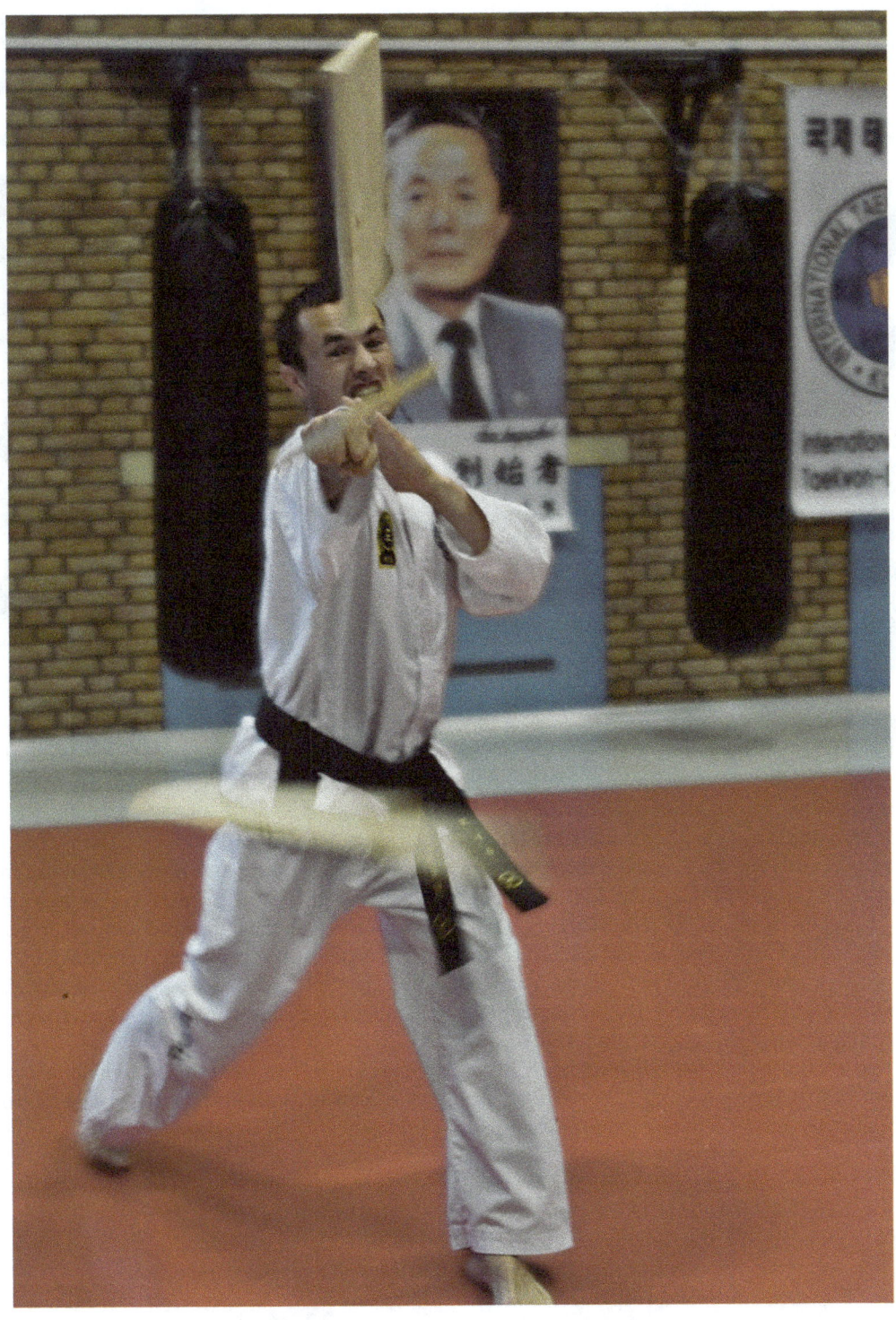

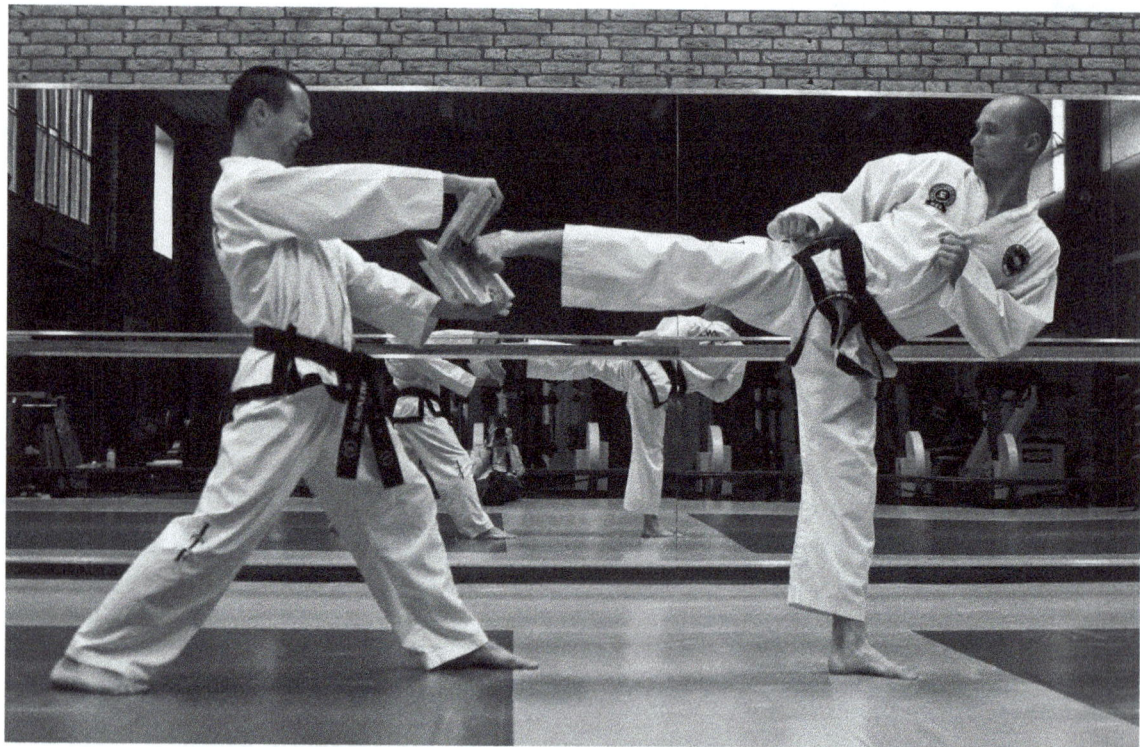

Precision and control break tests

With these types of break tests it is more about the speed and precision of a technique. These break tests require a great amount of control of the body and the technique. In general, spruce is the type of wood that is used for these tests. During grading examinations the board is loosely tied to a chain, which makes the point the force is focused on (the point of application) instable and therefore the board yields easier. The thickness of the board is determined according to the level of the student and the technique. Examples of precision and control break tests are breaking a board that is loosely hanging from a string, or breaking a board that one loosely holds or throws in the air themselves.

Until the 4th kub, break tests are generally executed on one or more plastic boards. During the grading exam, a wooden board that loosely hangs from a chain is used. From the 4th kub and up, during every grading exam one breaks with one hand technique and one foot technique. The exam committee determines how many boards one should break at once, and with which technique, depending on the level.

It is not sensible to use heavier breaking materials when performing break tests with younger children. The burden on the bones and joints of growing children is too heavy. However, there are many alternative materials and exercises to take some sort of test. Think of special plastic *youth* boards, for example.

There are certain conditions for making a break test as successful as possible, with a minimum chance of injuries:

- Correct execution;
- Hardening the body parts;
- Correct preparation;
- Mental relaxation and balance.

Correct execution

Technically, the technique must be perfect. One has to hit the material with the correct body part in the correct manner. The factors of strength development and strength control must be completely controlled. The smaller the surface of the point of contact on the body, the greater the effect will be. Even though all factors have their significance, speed and acceleration in the technique directed at the object that must be broken are the most important.

This is why a shorter and lighter person with a good technique can break as many objects as a taller or heavier person. All of the factors must create a complete, controlled, and devastating technique in harmony and consensus. This takes a lot of training.

Hardening the body parts

In Taekwon-Do, the body parts that are used for the break test must be hardened. When a body part is hardened, the chance of pain and possible injuries becomes smaller. There are several ways to harden body parts. For example, one can do pushups on the knuckles or fingertips instead of the hands. Also, one can hit one's own palm or execute a knife hand strike on the palm. As a means of practice, the forearms can be slammed together as well, with gradually increasing impact. In the Dojang, the impact of punches, strikes and kicks can be slowly increased; first on a punching bag, then on a Dallyon Joo, and finally on a brick wall. Hardening body parts asks much courage and perseverance of the student. Eventually, the nervous system will recognize this form of training, which will lessen the sensation of

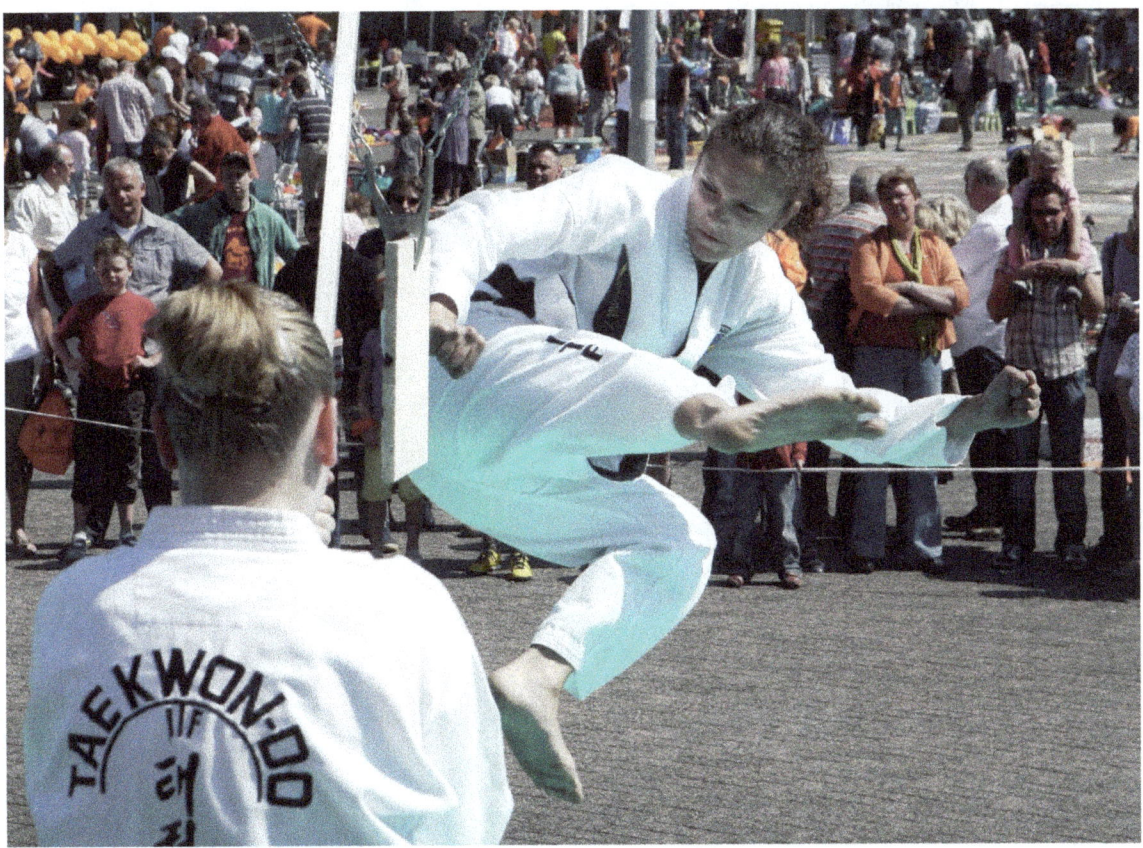

Boosabum Nadia Janssen 2th degree, student of the authors.

pain. Also, through this form of hardening the bone structure will become denser, making the bone harder and stronger.

Correct preparation
In this case, preparation for a break test is meant. Apart from the hardening, correct technique, and mental preparation, the test itself must be prepared as well. 'Which material will I be breaking? In what position am I in relation to the material that must be broken? How many degrees is the angle at which I will hit the material? Which part of the material will I hit? Which surface of my body part will make contact with the material? At which level should the material be held?' There are numerous elements that can be prepared in a break test. During exams, preparation is at times not taken seriously. This immediately decreases the chance of breaking the material.

Mental relaxation and balance
Ideally, the mind is empty; without thoughts such as fear of pain and failure. This is also called 'the indomitable mind'. Only then can body and mind be one, and can there be complete focus. The mental state of the Taekwon-Doin is of great importance. It is significant to have faith in one's own capacities as well as in the technique. When there is serious training, there will be self-confidence and a self-critical optimistic state of mind. At the moment of breaking, one will have an extraordinary sense of confidence, faith in oneself, and faith in the technique that is used. Because of the perception of success one will experience a sense of conviction and determination, which is absolutely important in becoming a good Taekwon-Do student. This is why break tests are an essential component of Taekwon-Do.

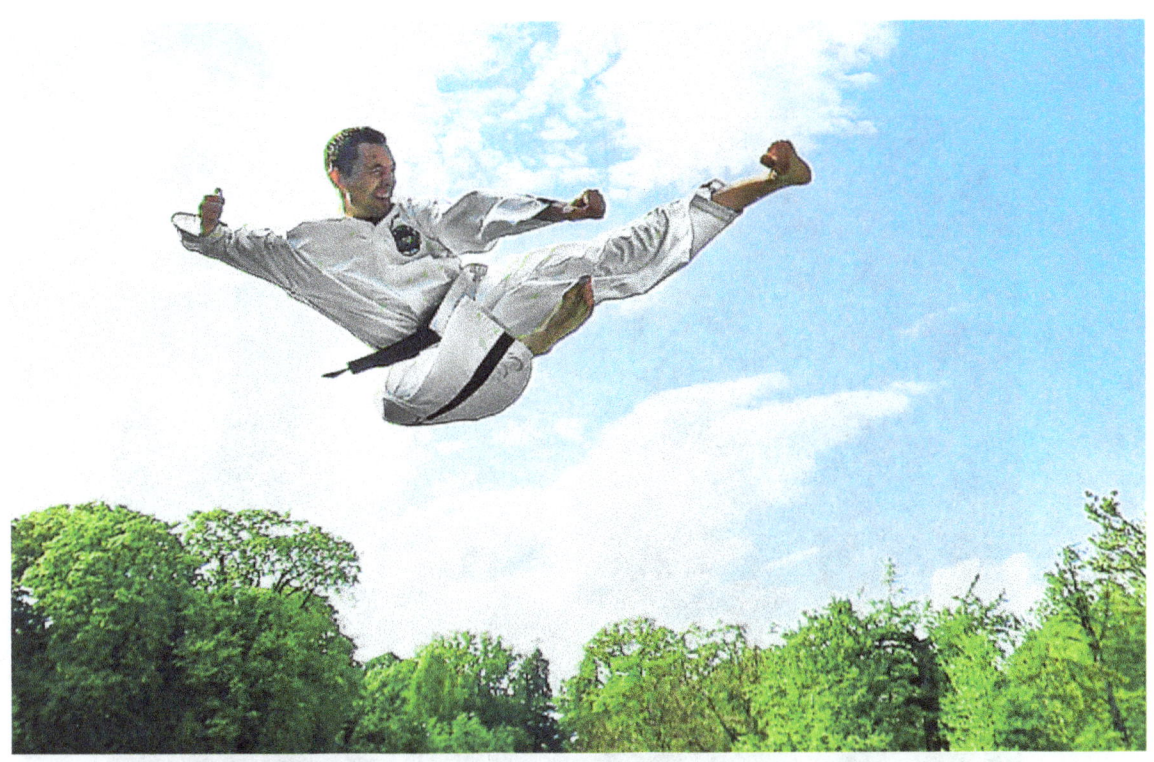
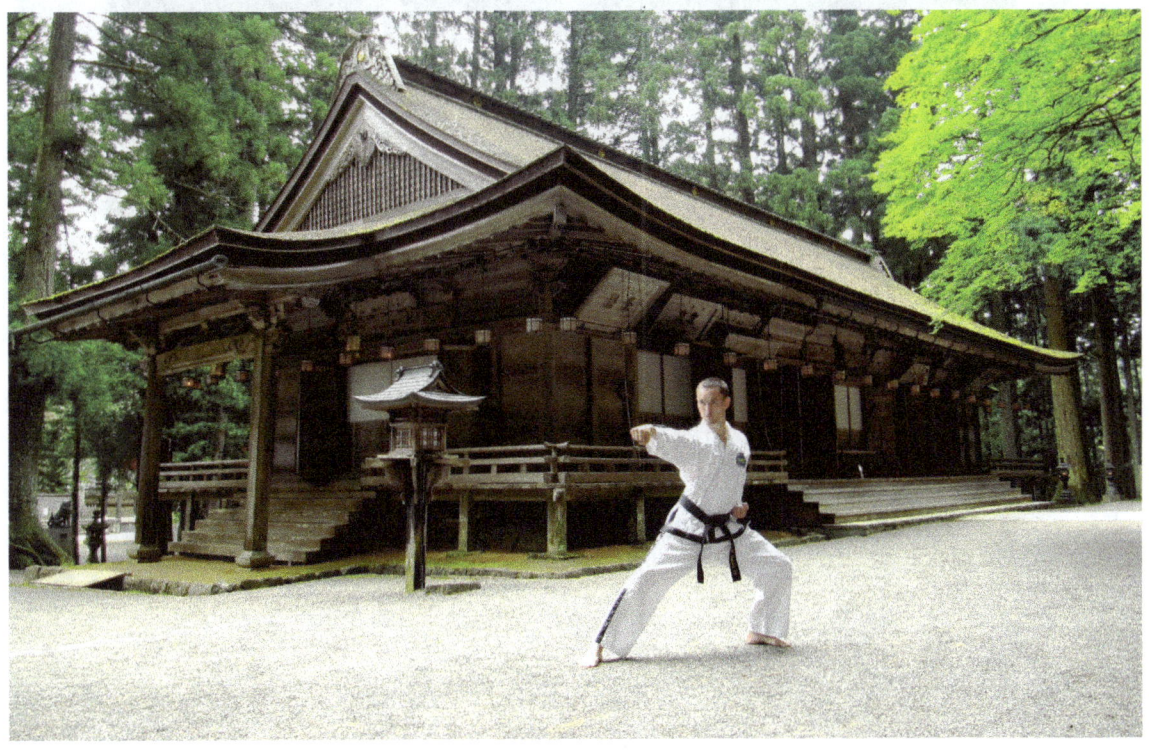

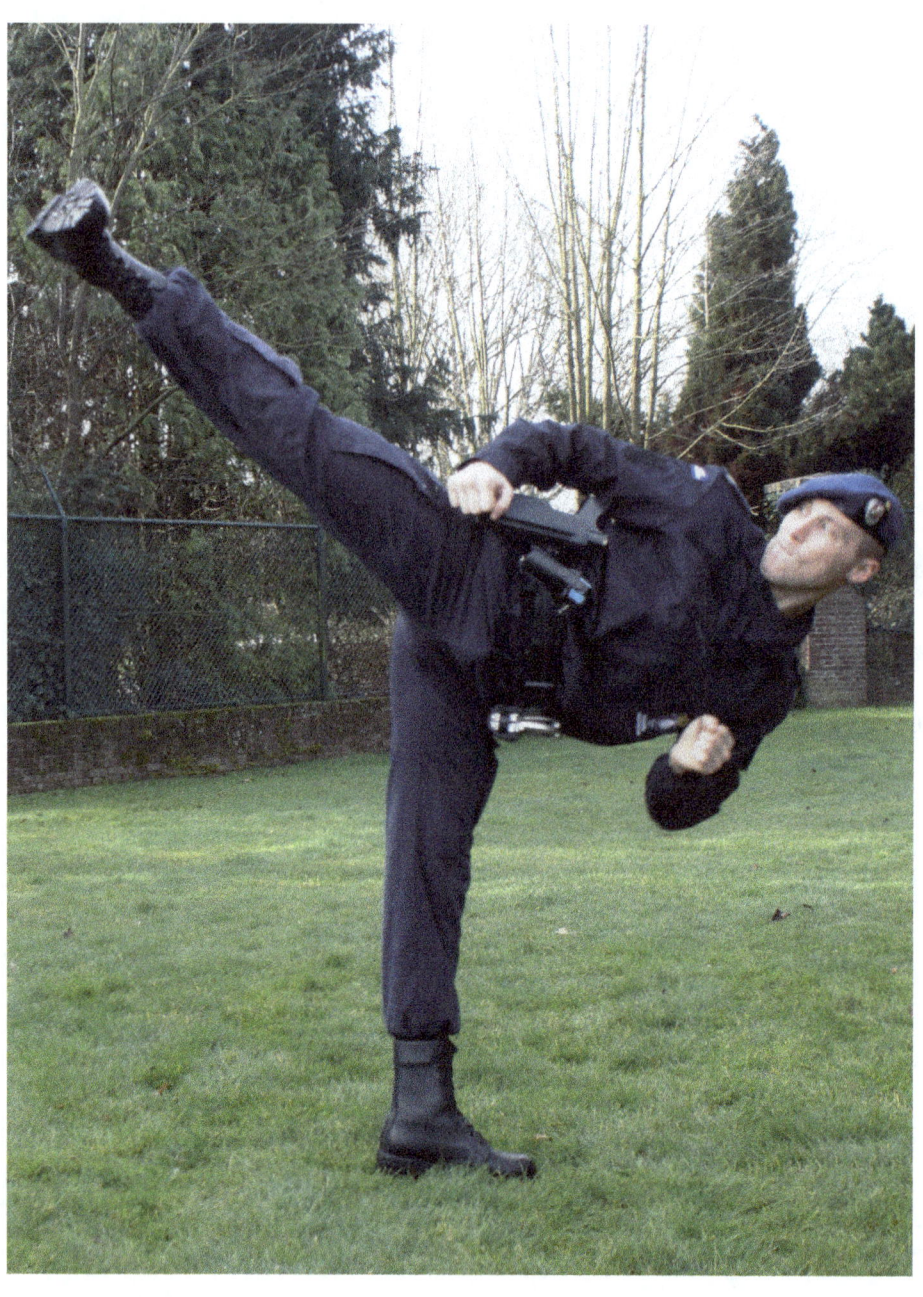

EPILOGUE

So much for the basics. Our goal was not just to discuss a number of essential matters, but also to clearly capture them in images. We wanted to clearly put the basic principles into words in order to clarify contemporary Taekwon-Do even more.

First and foremost, this book is meant as support and an addition to the regular training. The book does not replace the teacher or fellow student. Taekwon-Do must be physically practiced in order to possibly fully master it one day. The way of Taekwon-Do is a long way, which requires much effort and dedication. It is a way that presents different options for the person practicing Taekwon-Do. It is the way of the tuls and deepening, the way of sparring and competition, or a combination of it.

Either way, both the mind and the body will struggle at first to master the rich variety of techniques, let alone to understand the underlying philosophy. Our experience is that after a few years, the dedicated student will become increasingly proficient in Taekwon-Do.

For many, martial arts continue to be an almost bottomless well of energy, also in one's personal life. It is up to the motivated and disciplined student to grab every opportunity to become better at Taekwon-Do. It is your choice to be successful!

We sincerely hope the owner of this book has been able to broaden their vision and perspective, and has found an incentive to enrich themselves even more. This book is also an invitation to participate in the many regional and national training opportunities and seminars that the ITF Royal Dutch has to offer throughout the year.

For us, Taekwon-Do, the way of the foot and the fist, is
an art that goes beyond moving,
an art that brings people together,
an art that enhances physical strength,
an art that enhances mental determination,
an art that harmonizes body and spirit,
an art that stimulates courteousness, integrity, self-control, determination, and an invincible mind.

In short: Taekwon-Do, the Way to success!

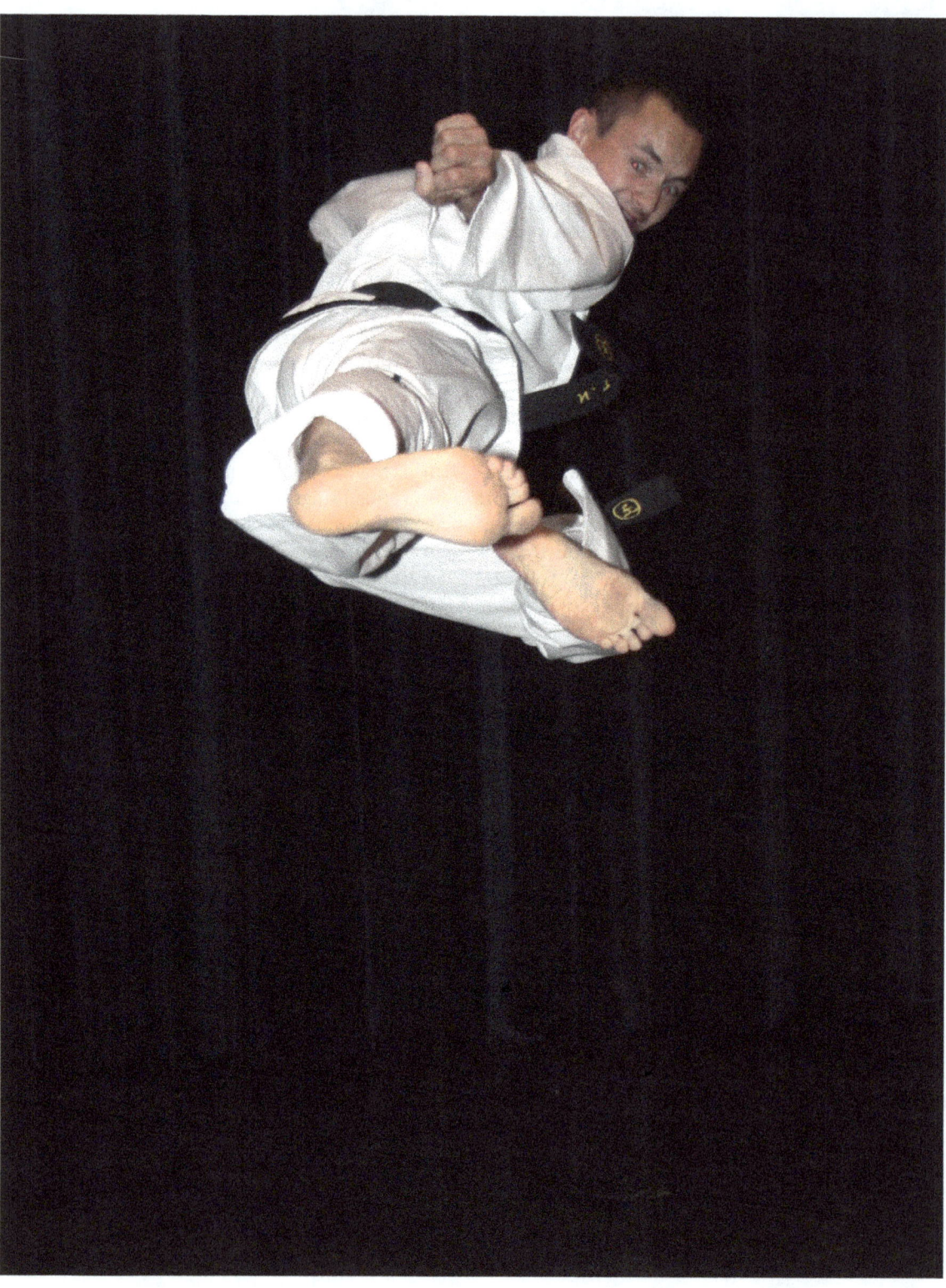

ACKNOWLEDGEMENTS

Many people have helped us to create this book, each of them in their own way. We are very grateful to all of them. We would specifically like to thank the following people.

A special thank you goes out to Martijn Koop. Through his editing and contributions to the text he has greatly contributed to this book. We also thank him for the hours of philosophizing about *martial arts* and its possibilities. Hopefully we will continue to inspire each other.

Thanks to Aron de Groot and Gert van Dam as well. Through our cooperation with them we have been able to add countless professional photographs and illustrations to the book. Thanks for their expertise, dedication, and above all their patience during the many hours of shooting.

A special thank you to Priscilla van Steen. Thank your for your input and support for the English version of this book. We couldn't have done it without you!

We would like to thank Master Zondag for his support while writing this book, and the inspiration he has been giving us for years. For us, every lesson is a mini-seminar.

We would like to thank President *Sabum* Thijssen for sharing his endless knowledge and his spiritual teachings. We are honored to be working on the board with these two mentors for the future of ITF Royal Dutch. We hope to be able to enjoy these incredible mentors for many years to come.

We would also like to thank *Sabum* Langeveld, with whom we have a special way of working and training together at ITF Royal Dutch.

We would like to thank the remaining members of the ITF Royal Dutch committee for their extraordinary input and dedication to the organization. Madam Ella Zondag, *Sabum* Dijkhuizen, *Sabum* Dekker, *Boosabum* van Dam, *Boosabum* Geijsberts, *Boosabum* Sleeuwenhoek and *Boosabum* Michon.

We want to thank the students and friends of Taekwon-Do Academie Gelderland for their constant enthusiasm and motivation. Specifically, we would like to thank *Boosabum* Burgers everything he has done for us. Furthermore, we want to thank our assistants, *Boosabum* Rikken, *Boosabum* Ripassa, and *Boosabum* Geleijnse for their loyal dedication to our academy.

We would also like to thank our international colleagues and Taekwon-Do friends. *Master* Nicolls and *Master* Skyrme from the United Kingdom, *Master* Maidana from Argentina, *Sabum* Braemer from Germany, *Master* Lee from Japan, and *Master* Cj-Oh and *Sabum* Sean-Yu from Korea. We would like to thank them for their friendship, hospitality, education, and the fine collaboration on an international level.

Also, we would like to take this opportunity to thank our parents for all the years of support. Since we were children, they have made it possible for us to chase our dreams, and they have created a fantastic foundation for us all these years.

Last, but certainly not least, we would like to thank Judith and Karen. For their understanding, appreciation, and especially the patience they have every time we engage in our other passion, week after week, and all over the world.

Taekwon!

PAUL VAN BEERSUM
WILLEM JANSEN

ABOUT THE AUTHORS

Paul van Beersum (1982)

Paul van Beersum was born in Elst, the Netherlands, on January 3rd, 1982. Van Beersum is an internationally acknowledged chief instructor of Taekwon-Do, an international ITF class 'A' referee, and in possession of the 4th dan in Taekwon-Do and the 1st dan in Hapkido.

At 13 years old van Beersum came into contact with Taekwon-Do at the Taekwon-Do School Bemmel, which was led by Herman Burgers. After two years he acquired his 1st dan in Taekwon-Do in 1997. After his high school years he started college at CIOS (Central Institute for the Education of Sports Instructors) in Arnhem. During this period of time, van Beersum came into contact with several Budo disciplines and was able to develop himself as a self-defense expert. In the meantime he remained passionate in practicing Taekwon-Do and was able to obtain several national titles on the highest level. Also, van Beersum was president of the national demonstration team. In 2002, van Beersum and Willem Jansen took over the Taekwon-Do school from Burgers. Since then, the school has been professionalized, with a new name as its most recent development: Taekwon-Do Academie Gelderland, TAG. In the meantime the school has delivered countless national champions and holders of dan ranks.

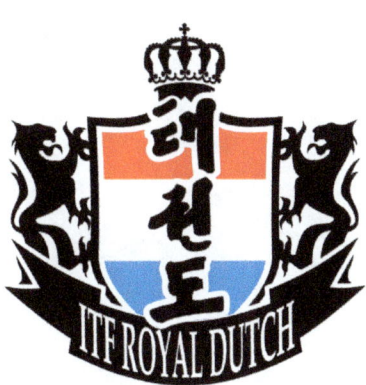

For a long time, van Beersum served as a sports instructor for the Royal Military Police. This has given him the opportunity to specialize in Arrest and Military Self-Defense Techniques. Van Beersum is a multiple National Military Judo Champion within the Ministry of Defense. During his term of national service he followed a part-time first degree physical education teaching program at the sports academy in Tilburg.

Currently, van Beersum works as a Sports and Movement teacher at Senior Secondary Vocational school ROC A12 in Velp, where he teaches students to become sports instructors or sports coordinators.

Van Beersum is co-founder and secretary of ITF Royal Dutch. Besides that, he is a national coach at the Committee of Technical Education. This team is responsible for the technical training sessions of the foundation, and consequently it is responsible for the technical level of Taekwon-Do in the Netherlands. Van Beersum follows international seminars with Taekwon-Do grandmasters in order to fulfill this task. In possession of a first degree teaching certificate, van Beersum teaches classes for the Teacher Training College Committee which are aimed at training students so that they will be able to give didactical, pedagogical and psychologically responsibly Taekwon-Do lessons.

Willem Jansen (1979)

Willem Jansen was born in Nijmegen, the Netherlands, on June 5th, 1979. He is an internationally acknowledged chief instructor of Taekwon-Do, an international ITF class 'A' referee, and in possession of the 4th dan in Taekwon-Do and the 1st dan in Hapkido.

At the age of 13, Jansen started practicing Taekwon-Do at Taekwon-Do Academy Taekyon in Bemmel. After two years, he obtained his 1st dan in Taekwon-Do in 1995. During his high school years in Bemmel, Jansen acquired his assistant-instructor's certificate. He moved to Tilburg for his studies and graduated from the Academy for Physical Education in 2002, as a first degree physical education instructor and a sports masseur.

During his time at the Academy, Jansen came into contact with several Budo disciplines. He also remained active in Taekwon-Do and acquired several national titles at the highest level. Jansen was a member of the national demonstration team as well. In Tilburg he successfully introduced Taekwon-Do to the student sports center of the University of Tilburg and independently taught Taekwon-Do lessons to students. In 2002, Jansen and van Beersum took over the Taekwon-Do School Bemmel.

Since 2002, Jansen has been teaching physical education at the Olympus College in Arnhem, where he is also president of the physical education department. For this department Jansen has been responsible for the construction of the sports center, fitness center, and Dojang. Through his initiative, Taekwon-Do and self-defense have been added to the school's curriculum. This makes the Olympus College the first high school for secondary education in the Netherlands that has Taekwon-Do on its curriculum. The school Dojang is unique in its kind for high schools in the Netherlands.

Jansen is co-founder and board member of the ITF Royal Dutch. Besides that, he is a national coach and president of the Committee of Technical Education of the ITF Royal Dutch. Also, he is an instructor for and member of the Teacher Training College Committee.

Aside from Taekwon-Do, Jansen has another passion, which is travelling the countries where the roots of Asian martial arts lie. During his travels through Asia (Korea, Japan, China, Vietnam, Cambodia, Indonesia, and Thailand) he always attempts to stay at Buddhist temples and to come into contact with local martial artists.

APPENDIX I
GLOSSARY OF KOREAN WORDS AND DEFINITIONS

Since Taekwon-Do is a Korean martial art, the authors have used Korean terms in this book. Every Taekwon-Do student should work with Korean terms from the very beginning. Eventually, one should know the Korean names for the most important basic and fundamental exercises. Using these terms creates more depth and (inter)national unity. After all, through the use of Korean nomenclature it is possible to communicate with Taekwon-Do colleagues from all over the world.

Korean is partially derived from Chinese. 'Hangul' is the Korean script used to write the Korean language. 'Hangul' is alphabetic and phonetic. It consists of 28 characters, of which 24 are used. Therefore it is relatively easy to learn. Since the language is phonetic, much attention has to be paid to how to pronounce the words. If a word has a different sound, it probably also has a different meaning. Throughout time, 'Hangul' has been adapted to the Roman language. For example, the 'Ch'-sound has become a 'J'-sound, creating Jeju instead of Cheju.

The authors feel that every Taekwon-Do student needs to become acquainted with the Korean terms from the first encounter with Taekwon-Do. Next is a list of the Korean terms, with their English definitions, that can be found up to the 1st dan.

Stances
charyot	– being in position
ke	– face toward
kyongye	– extend greeting
junbi	– ready stance
si jak	– start
guman	– stop
swiyo	– relax in parallel ready stance
hae san	– send away

Dojang and surroundings
dojang	– training space (the place where 'the way' is practiced)
Han-guk	– Korea
kuryung e machuoso	– with command (on count)
kuryung obsi	– without command
dobok	– Taekwon-Do attire
ti	– belt
kupso	– vital parts
gi	– energy or inner (life) strength
jeja	– student
boosabum (nim)	– assistant instructor (1st to 3rd dan)
sabum (nim)	– instructor (4th to 6th dan)
sahyun (nim)	– master (7th to 8th dan)
saseong (nim)	– grandmaster (9th dan)
changnika (nim)	– founder
nim	– respected

General terms
makgi	– block
jirugi	– punch
taerigi	– strike
tulgi	– thrust
chagi	– kick
kye pa	– break test

hosinsul	– self-defense	bandea	– opposite
mong nyom	– meditation	baro	– direct (technique on the leg side that is bent most)

Body parts

sondabak	– palm	doo	– double
sonkal	– knife hand	sang	– twin
sonkut	– fingertips		

Stances

sonkal dung	– inner knife hand
palmok	– forearm
an palmok	– inner forearm
bakat palmok	– outer forearm
dung joomuk	– back fist
joomuk	– fist
songarak joomuk	– knuckle fist
yop joomuk	– side fist
palkup	– elbow
dwit kumchi	– back sole
dwichook	– back heel
balkal	– side heel
baldung	– instep
apkumchi	– ball of foot
moorup	– knee

niunja sogi	– L-stance
gojung sogi	– fixed L-stance
gunnun sogi	– walking stance
nachuo sogi	– fixed walking stance
annun sogi	– sitting stance
kyocha sogi	– X-stance
waebal sogi	– one-leg stance
dwitbal sogi	– rear foot stance
moa sogi	– close stance
narani sogi	– parallel stance
guburyo sogi	– bending stance
junbi sogi	– ready stance
soojik sogi	– vertical stance

Classification of techniques

bang eo gi	– defensive techniques
gong gyuk gi	– attacking techniques
soo gi	– hand techniques
jok gi	– foot techniques

Directions and heights

wen	– left
orun	– right
najunde	– low
kaunde	– middle
nopunde	– high
ap	– front
dwit	– reverse
yop	– side
dollyo	– turning
anuro	– inward
bakuro	– outward
naeryo	– downward
chookyo	– rising
ollyo	– upward
sewo	– vertical
soopyong	– horizontal
an	– inner
bakat	– outer
pihagi	– evade
twiro tora	– turn
kiokja	– angle

Techniques up to the 1st dan

Punching techniques

ap joomuk jirugi	– forefist punch
bandae ap joomuk jirugi	– front forefist reverse punch
yop jirugi	– side fist punch
sang soomuk sewo jirugi	– twin forefist vertical punch
sang joomuk dwijibo jirugi	– twin fist upset punch
giokja jirugi	– angle punch
baro ollyo jirugi	– obverse upward punch

Thrusting techniques

sun sonkut tulgi	– straight fingertip thrust
dwijibun sonkut tulgi	– upset fingertip thrust

sang yop palkup tulgi – twin side elbow thrust
opun sonkut tulgi – flat fingertip thrust (palm downward)
yop palkup tulgi – side elbow thrust

Striking techniques
sonkal bakuro taerigi – outward knife hand strike
sonkal yop taerigi – knife hand side strike
sonkal anuro taerigi – inward knife hand strike
ap palkup bandae taerigi – reverse front elbow strike
dung joomuk yop taerigi – back fist side strike
wi palkup bandae taerigi – reverse upper elbow strike
dung joomuk yopdwi taerigi – back fist side back strike
sonkal naeryo taerigi – downward knife hand strike
sonkal dung ap taerigi – front reverse knife hand strike

Foot techniques
ap chagi – front kick
ap chagi busigi – front snap kick
cha busigi – snap kick
yop chagi jirugi – side piercing kick
yopcha tulgi – side thrusting kick
yopcha milgi – side pushing kick
yopcha momchugi – side checking kick
dollyo chagi – turning kick
dwit chagi jirugi – back piercing kick
sewo chagi – vertical kick
suroh chagi – sweeping kick
golcho chagi – hooking kick
noollo chagi – pressing kick
bandal chagi – crescent kick
bandae dollyo goro chagi – reverse hooking kick
bandae dollyo chagi – reverse turning kick
naeryo chagi – downward kick
moorup ollyo chagi – knee upward kick
bituro chagi – twisting kick
twimyo chagi – flying kick

Blocks
noollo makgi – pressing block
miro makgi – pushing block
momchau makgi – checking block
daebi makgi – guarding block
dollimyo makgi – circular block
golcho makgi – hooking block
hechyo makgi – wedging block
chookyo makgi – rising block
kyocha makgi – X-fist block
sondabak makgi – palm block
digutja makgi – U-shape block
san makgi – W-shape block
sonkal makgi – knife hand block
sonkal dung makgi – reverse knife hand block
bakat palmok makgi – outside forearm block
anpalmok makgi – inner forearm block
anpalmok ap makgi – front inner forearm block
sondabak ollyo makgi – palm upward block
doo palmok makgi – double forearm block
daebi makgi – guarding block
sonkal daebi makgi – knife hand guarding block
palmok daebi makgi – forearm guarding block
anpalmok dollimyo makgi – inner circular block
sondabak golcho makgi – palm hooking block
sondabak bandae noollo makgi – palm pressing block
sang palmok makgi – twin forearm block
sang sonkal makgi – twin knife hand block
sang sondabak makgi – twin palm block (downward)
sang sondabak ollyo makgi – twin palm upward block
kyocha joomuk chookyo makgi – X-fist rising block
doo palmok miro makgi – double forearm pushing block
sondabak miro makgi – palm pushing block
kyocha sonkal momchau makgi – X-knife hand checking block
anpalmok yobap – inner forearm side front

makgi	block	8th	– pal
kyocha joomuk noollo makgi	– X-fist pressing block	9th	– koo
		10th	– shib
bakat palmok hechyo makgi	– outer forearm wedging block	**Tuls**	
		Chon-Ji	– 1
bakat palmok san makgi	– outer forearm W-shape block	Dan-Gun	– 2
		Do-San	– 3
		Won-Hyo	– 4
Sparring exercises		Yul-Gok	– 5
ilbo matsogi	– 1-step sparring	Joong-Gun	– 6
ibo matsogi	– 2-step sparring	Toi-Gye	– 7
ban jayoo matsogi	– semi-free sparring	Hwa-Rang	– 8
jok gi matsogi	– foot sparring	Choong-Moo	– 9
jayoo matsogi	– free sparring	Kwang-Gae	– 10
		Po-Eun	– 11
General competition terms		Ge-Baek	– 12
kam yom hana	– penalty point deduction	Eui-Am	– 13
kyungo hana	– warning	Chong-Jang	– 14
hye chyo	– stop	Ju-Che	– 15
hong	– red	Sam-Il	– 16
chong	– blue	Yoo-Sin	– 17
chida	– loser	Choi-Young	– 18
sung	– winner	Yon-Gae	– 19
mu-sung	– undecided	Ul-Ji	– 20
		Moon-Moo	– 21
Counting		So-San	– 22
1	– hana	Se-Jong	– 23
2	– dool	Tong-Il	– 24
3	– set		
4	– net		
5	– tasut		
6	– yausut		
7	– ilgope		
8	– yaudul		
9	– ahope		
10	– yaul		
1st	– ill		
2nd	– yee		
3th	– sam		
4th	– sah		
5th	– oh		
6th	– yook		
7th	– chil		

APPENDIX 2
GENERAL OVERVIEW OF DEFINITIONS

In Appendix 1 the basic Korean words and terms have been clarified. Next, the remaining words and terms that can be found in this book will be explained.

Aikido Japanese martial art that was developed by O-Sensei Morihei Ueshiba.

Bodhidarma Indian monk who taught zen meditation and martial arts at the Chinese shaolin monastery. In China he is known as Do Mo, and in Japan as Duruma.

Buddhism Religion that spread through East-Asia from India. Within Buddhism, there are many different directions. Buddhism has had a great influence in the development of martial arts.

Bruce Lee Chinese philosopher, martial artist, and movie star. Founder of Jeet Kune Do, passed away at the age of 32 (1973).

Budo Collective term for (Japanese) martial arts.

Chakras Energy fields in the human body. There are 7 main chakras.

Chang-Hun Choi Hong Hi's pseudonym as well as the name of his style of Taekwon-Do.

Chi Chinese term for energy or inner (life) strength.

Choi Hong Hi Founder of Taekwon-Do. Born in the Hwa Dae, Myong Chun district (1918-2002).

Choi Jung Hwa Son of the founder of Taekwon-Do (born in South Korea, 1954). President of the International Taekwon-Do Federation (ITF). Grandmaster (9th dan) in Taekwon-Do.

Confucius Chinese scholar (551-479 B.C.). His philosophy is based on inner virtues such as humanity and justice.

Dan Degree or rank for advanced students.

Do Method, way (of life). Martial arts that use the term 'Do' strive for character shaping of the student next to technical skills.

Eum-Yang Korean name for yin-yang. The Korean flag has the colors red-blue; red stands for yang (positive) and blue stands for eum (negative).

Fundamental exercises Fundamental exercises are the foundation of Taekwon-Do. They can be divided into: stances, walking techniques, hand techniques, foot techniques, and breathing exercises. They are applied in many forms, such as the tuls, partner exercises, break tests, etc.

Gi	Korean term for energy or inner (life) strength.		ITF Taekwon-Do in all its aspects, to everyone. The founders of ITF Royal Dutch are Master Zondag, Sabum Thijssen, Sabum van Beersum, and Sabum Jansen.
Gichin Funakoshi	Founder of the modern (Shotokan) Karate-do (1869-1957).		
Hae Dong Gumdo	Korean martial art that uses sword techniques that originate from the battlefield.	**Jeet Kune Do**	Martial art that was developed by Bruce Lee. Literally means 'The way of the Intercepting Fist'. This style is based on Lee's philosophy.
Hammudo	Korean martial art, is very similar to Hapkido.	**Jiu Jitsu**	Japanese martial art of elimination.
Han-Il Dong	Korean master in calligraphy and T'aekkyŏn.	**Judo**	Japanese martial art. Literally means 'the soft way', developed by professor Jigoro Kano in 1882. Judo is derived from Jiu Jitsu and was developed for education.
Hapkido	Korean art of self-defense. It is derived from several different traditional martial arts, such as Japanese Daito Ryu Aiki Jutsu. It is based on the harmony of mental and physical strength. Characteristic for Hapkido are the self-defense techniques where one uses the strength of the opponent.	**Karate**	Also known as Karate-Do. Japanese martial art, which literally means 'empty hand' or 'hand of China', depending on how it is written.
		Kata	Japanese term for 'form'. A series of techniques based on imaginary opponents, which was arranged in advance.
Hwarang-do	Korean art of self-defense and art of medicine.		
ITF	International Taekwon-Do Federation. After the death of the founder it was split into 3 world organizations. The ITF Royal Dutch is affiliated with the ITF of Grandmaster Choi Jung Hwa.	**Kendo**	'The way of the sword'. Japanese sword art. One uses a bamboo stick, which represents a long sword.
		Ki	Japanese term for energy or inner (life) strength.
ITF Royal Dutch	Dutch national foundation that was founded in Bunnik on February 3rd, 2010 and affiliated with world organization ITF of Grandmaster Choi Jung Hwa. One of the objectives of the foundation is to promote traditional	**KTA**	Korean Taekwon-Do Association.
		Kub	Grade or rank for beginners.
		Kuk Sool Won	Korean art of self-defense developed by master Suh In Huyk.

	Self-defense, meditation, and chi are crucial.		1965 by Dutch judo instructor Wagner. He has intensively promoted Taekwon-Do in the Netherlands until 1968. After that, he moved to Canada where he still teaches Taekwon-Do.
Kum-do	Korean sword art. Literally means 'the way of the sword'.		
Kung Fu	Collective term for different Chinese martial arts, forms of acrobatics, forms of movement and forms of medicine. In China, this is called Wushu.	**Poomsae**	WTF Taekwon-Do (style) figures. There are 17 style figures and they are called taegeuk. Taegeuk 1 through 8 are for those in possession of the kubs.
Kwan	Korean term for house or school.	**Saju Jirugi**	Preparatory tul, 'four directional punch'.
Kwon Moo Gun	Korean who studied medicine in Germany and who was introduced Taekwon-Do in the Netherlands (invited by judo instructor Hendriks from Venlo). In 1968 he returned to Korea.	**Saju Makgi**	Preparatory tul, 'four directional defense'.
		Shaolin temple	Chinese temple in the Henan province, where the hard style of Chinese martial arts and Zen Buddhism were developed.
Lao Zi	Founder of Taoism. Lived in China in the 6th century B.C.		
Meridians	Paths that according to traditional Chinese medicine circulate energy through the body. These paths are connected to each other.	**Shotokan**	Style of karate developed in Okinawa by Funakoshi around the 1920s.
		Subak	Ancient lost Korean martial art.
Mudo	Korean term for martial arts.	**Taegeuk**	See Poomsae.
Nam Tae Hi	Associate of Choi Hong Hi and Taekwon-Do pioneer from the first hour.	**Taegeukgi**	Name of the Korean flag.
		Taeguk	Korean name for the Taoist circle of Eum-Yang.
Newton	Sir Isaac Newton (1643-1727). English scholar and founder of classical mechanics.	**Taekwon-Doin**	Practitioner of Taekwon-Do.
Oh Do Kwan	'Training my way'. The name of the military academy of Choi Hong Hi.	**T'aekkyŏn**	Old Korean martial art of unarmed fighting, where the focus is on leg techniques and the objective is to make the opponent lose their balance. Since recently T'aekkyŏn has been blossoming
Park Jong Soo	Korean Taekwon-Do master, brought to the Netherlands in		

in South-Korea.

Tai Chi (Chuan) Chinese inner martial art. Characteristic are the soft and flowing motions. Tai Chi is also knows as shadow boxing. Literally means 'supreme ultimate fist'.

Tang Soo Do Korean martial art. Literally means 'the art of the Tang hand'. Tang can also be read as 'China', which would change the meaning to 'the art of the Chinese hand'. Tang Soo Do has many Japanese Shotokan Karate influences.

Tao The Way or path in Chinese (also known as Dao).

Taoism A Chinese philosophy. Based on the traditional concept of Yin-Yang and Chi. This religion encourages following one's intuition, nature, and the Way (Do, or Tao in Chinese). Also see Lao Zi.

Vital spots Locations or places on or inside the body that can be fatally injured when hit in the correct spot. The body has hundreds of vital spots.

Yin-Yang Chinese principle of duality. Based on cooperating and counteracting forces. 'Yang' represents 'positive' and 'Yin' stands for the opposite, 'negative'. Together they form the Taoist vision of the universe.

Yoga Indian philosophy and styles of meditation and positions.

WTF World Taekwon-do Federation. Founded in 1973. The WTF style, practice forms, and sparring rules have little in common with ITF Taekwon-Do. The WTF style mainly focuses on Taekwon-Do as (competitive) sport.

Zen Buddhist philosophy of meditation and an attitude to life in order to reach enlightenment. The philosophy of tranquility.

APPENDIX 3
INTERPRETATION OF THE EMBLEM OF TAEKWON-DO ACADEMIE GELDERLAND (TAG)

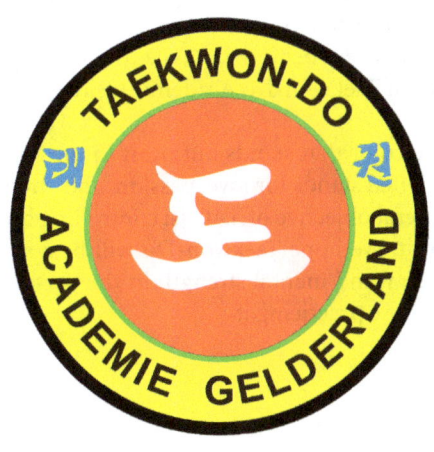

The emblem of Taekwon-Do Academie Gelderland

1. The TAG emblem is round. This symbolizes the path of Taekwon-Do. This path fundamentally is a cycle. In this cycle, the Taekwon-Do student encounters multiple interesting elements (fundamental exercises, tuls, sparring, break tests, self-defense, esoteric exercises, and more). One starts practicing the martial art Taekwon-Do, and basically there is no end. If one thinks the end is in sight, a new challenge will cross their paths somehow. The same principle applies to acquiring the 1st dan; after that, one starts over.

2. The black frame of the emblem symbolizes the elegance a Taekwon-Doin should emanate.
Also, the black frame represents the universe. The universe is enormous, similar to the full knowledge of Taekwon-Do.

3. The outer circle contains the name of the school, in which:

- Taekwon-Do stands for a Korean way of unarmed fighting and mental training. Arms and legs are used for blocks, evasions, punches and kicks with the goal of quickly eliminating the opponent(s). Taekwon-Do techniques are based on modern physics. However, Taekwon-Do is more than a way of fighting. This is because of the personal philosophy of the founder and the Do that is so strongly represented in traditional Taekwon-Do. The term Do is difficult to explain sometimes, especially for the Western frame of mind. Do is more than just a method. Do is a traditional way of life from East-Asia. It consists of living with a good life attitude or mental attitude. It is very significant how one walks the way. In that sense, Taekwon-Do is a way of life. Think of Taekwon-Do as health exercise for body and spirit, the pedagogic value of Taekwon-Do, or learning to defend oneself.

- Academy stands for university or educational institute. TAG is an Academy for any serious martial artist who strives to achieve their maximum potential, and where martial arts are taught and studied at a high level. Academy also stands for the general level of training of its instructors. The main instructors have their 1st degree for teaching physical education at elementary schools, high schools, and in higher education, next to the Taekwon-Do specific required teacher and referee acknowledgements.

- The province of Gelderland symbolizes the history as well as the ambition of TAG. The village of Bemmel, located in Gelderland, is where in the 1970s the foundation for the Academy was created at the Taekwon-Do School Bemmel. Furthermore, Gelderland stands for the members and range of the academy. Today, Taekwon-Do students from outside the village and even province are attending the schools of TAG to learn the art of Taekwon-Do. The ambition of TAG is to become a nationally acknowledged academy, with international respectability.

4. The emblem has the colors of all developmental stages of a Taekwon-Do student:

   White is the color of innocence: the beginning student has no prior knowledge of Taekwon-Do.
   Yellow is the color of the earth: a plant sprouts and roots itself, such as the student that is acquiring the basics of Taekwon-Do.
   Green is the color of the plant, that grows and develops itself. The student is starting to develop itself in the art of Taekwon-Do.
   Blue is the color of the sky, to which the plant ripens itself. In a similar way, the student develops itself through practice.
   Red is the color of danger, which warns the student to stay in control, and also warns the adversary to stay away.
   Black is the opposite of white. Therefore, it signifies the *ripeness* and *skill* in Taekwon-Do.

5. The blue Korean symbols represent 'Tae' (the foot) and 'Kwon' (the fist). Almost all defense and attack techniques are executed with the four limbs. Together, 'Tae' and 'Kwon' – 'Taekwon' – represent the international Taekwon-Do greeting for respect and appreciation.

6. The great white Korean symbol or character ('Do') represents the way of life and the art. The way of Taekwon-Do stands for the way that leads to becoming a pure person, which consists of 5 fundamental principles. These are the moral values that Taekwon-Do is based upon:

   - Ye Ui: Courtesy & politeness
   - Yom Chi: Integrity & honesty
   - In Nae: Persistance & patience
   - Guk Gi: Self-control
   - Baekjool Boolgool: Invincible spirit

   The 'Do' symbol is deliberately centered in the emblem. The 'Do' symbol is white, which stands for peace, purity, innocence, and an empty mind. The concept behind 'Do' is central in the philosophy of Taekwon-Do Academie Gelderland.

7. The color that stands out most in the emblem is red. Red stands for love, passion, and energy. The general objective of TAG is: controlling body and spirit. We hope Taekwon-Do will be a source of energy and mental strength in the personal lives of those practicing it.

APPENDIX 4
RECOMMENDED AND CONSULTED LITERATURE

Bax, Hilde & Heuvel, Anton van den (1999)
Ethiek in beweging, Bewegen en ethiek in onderwijs, sport en gezondheidscentra.
Assen, Nederland: Van Gorcum

Brennran, Barbara Ann (2005)
Bronnen van licht. Haarlem, Nederland: Altamira-Brecht.

Bloem, Jan & Hoorn, Rob van der (2004)
Opvoeden op de mat, over opvoedkundige waarde van stoei- en trefsporten. IOS-project 'krachten bundelen' i.s.m. Landelijk samenwerkingsverband 'Sportiviteit en Respect'.

Boersma, W. & Edel, M. den (1999)
Jiu-Jitsu do. Rijswijk, Nederland: Elmar.

Choi, Hong Hi (1998)
Taekwon-Do. The Korean Art of Self-Defence. Canada: International Taekwon-Do Federation.

Choi, Hong Hi (1993)
Encyclopedia of Taekwon-Do. Mississauga, Canada: International Taekwon-Do Federation.

Choi, Hong Hi
Taekwon-Do and I. The memoirs of Choi Hong Hi, the founder of Taekwon-Do.
Mississauga, Canada: International Taekwon-Do Federation.

Choi, Hong Hi
Moral Guide Book. Mississauga, Canada: International Taekwon-Do Federation.

Chong, Lee (1975)
Dynamic kicks, essentials for free fighting. Burbank, California, V.S.: Ohara.

Chong, Lee (1978)
Advanced explosive kicks. Santa Clarita, California, V.S.: Ohara.

Cho, Hee Il (1981)
Man of contrasts. Los Angeles, V.S.: Hee Il Cho.

De Koop, Scheerder en Vanreusel (2006)
Sportsociologie, het spel en de spelers. Maarssen, Nederland: Elsevier gezondheidszorg.

Holvast, H (1977)
Taekwondo, Steenwijk, Nederland: Hovens Gréve

Hu, Bin (1991)
Keep fit the Chinese way. Beijing, China: Foreign Languages Press.

Hyams, Joe (1979)
Zen in the martial arts. New York, V.S.: Bantam.

Kelch, Alexander (1991)
Bruchtests, taekwondo in perfection. Niedernhausen, Duitsland: Falken.

Kruyning, Edgar (2002)
Dynamic budo/1 De Yoseikan spirit. Rijswijk, Nederland: Elmar.

Lam, Kam Chuen (2003)
Da cheng chuan, oefeningen voor het vergroten van innerlijke kracht. Haarlem, Nederland: Altamira-Becht.

Lee, Bruce (1975)
Tao of Jeet Kune Do. Burbank, California, V.S.: Ohara.

Lee, Bruce & Little, John (1998)
The art of expressing the human body. North Clarendon, Vermont, Canada: Tuttle.

Meertens & Grumbow (1992)
Sociale Psychologie. Groningen, Nederland: Wolters Noordhoff.

Mietzel, G. (1988)
Wegwijs in psychologie, psychologie voor de praktijk, Zutphen, Nederland: Thieme.

Mitchell, David (1985)
Alles over vechtsporten. Utrecht, Nederland: Kosmos.

Miyamoto, Musashi (2001)
Het boek van de vijf ringen. Haarlem, Nederland: Altamira-Brecht.

Molen, IJ.van der (1994)
Opvoedingstheorie en opvoedingspraktijk. Groningen, Nederland: Wolters Norrdhoff

Nonanchuk, T.A. & MacNeil, M.C. (1989)
Examinations of the effects of traditional martial art training on aggressiveness.
In: Human Relations, June Vol. 34 (6).

Orschouw, K. van & Teeuwissen, J. & Oeveren, S. van (1998-2004)
Werkboek Taekwon-do, Nederland: United taekwondo International (3 delen).

Reid, Howard & Croucher, Michael (1983)
The Way of the Warrior, The Paradox of the Martial Arts. Woodstock, New York, V.S.: The Overlook Press.

Sharamon & Baginski (1990)
Het chakra handboek. Amsterdam, Nederland: Boekschors.

Sleijfer, J.A. (2005)
Vechtsport maakt jongens wel/niet agressief. In: Lichamelijke Opvoeding. KVLO: nr. 14, jaargang 93.

Suh, In Hyuk (1988)
Kuk Sool Won, breaking techniques. Pusan, Korea: Sport Life Publication.

Tedeschi, Marc (2000)
Hapkido: traditions, philosophy, technique. Boston, V.S.: Weatherhill.

Tedeschi, Marc (2000)
Essential Anatomy for Martial and Healing Arts. Boston, V.S.: Weatherhill.

Thoutenhoofd, Rien (1987)
Tae kwon do, theorie en praktijk
Rijswijk, Nederland: Elmar

Tohei, Koichi (1995)
Ki in het dagelijks leven. Haarlem, Nederland: Altamira-Brecht.

Weinmann, Wolfgang (1987)
Lexicon van de martial arts, Rijswijk, Nederland: Elmar

Wong, Kiew Kit (2001)
Handboek Tai-Chi Chuan. Utrecht, Nederland: Kosmos.

APPENDIX 5
USEFUL ADDRESSES AND WEBSITES

Taekwon-Do organizations

ITF Royal Dutch
Sterrenlaan 67
2402 AT Alphen a/d Rijn
Phone: +31 172 422335
E-mail: secretariaat@itf-royaldutch.com
Website: www.itf-royaldutch.com

ITF
International Taekwon-Do Federation
Yiewsley Leisure Centre
Otterfield Road, Yiewsley
United Kingdom
Phone: +44 1895 427356
E-mail: secgen@itf-administration.com
Website: www.itf-administration.com

More information on the internet

www.itf-royaldutch.com
www.taekwon-do.nl
www.itf-administration.com
www.itfline.org
www.tagelderland.nl

Contact information

For additional information or to get in touch with the authors, you can reach them by email at info@tagelderland.nl or you can take a look at their website: www.tagelderland.nl. If you are planning to visit the Netherlands you are more than welcome to join a class or take a private lesson with the authors.

APPENDIX 6
ITF PATTERN INSTRUCTION CARDS

These instruction cards can serve different purposes. They are ideal as a learning tool for new skills, but can also be used for quick revision on acquired skills.

Also, instructors can use them during lessons (competence aimed education).

Furthermore, students can use them as a reference card to practise or refresh their skills in a quick and effective manner. Last but not least: they are a great decoration for your Dojang!

With the approval of ITF Royal Dutch, these cards contain:
- The Korean names of all the patterns that the students need know
- All pattern techniques a student has to master
- The correct direction in which the techniques must be performed by the student
- The philosophical background of the pattern the student needs to know
- The diagram which symbolizes the pattern
- The colour of the card is linked to the different grades of coloured belts

This series of 9 IC cards in English have been developed from Chon-Ji up to Choong-Moo (patterns 1-9).

Printed on solid paper for excellent quality.

Order from www.tagelderland.nl and fill out the form.

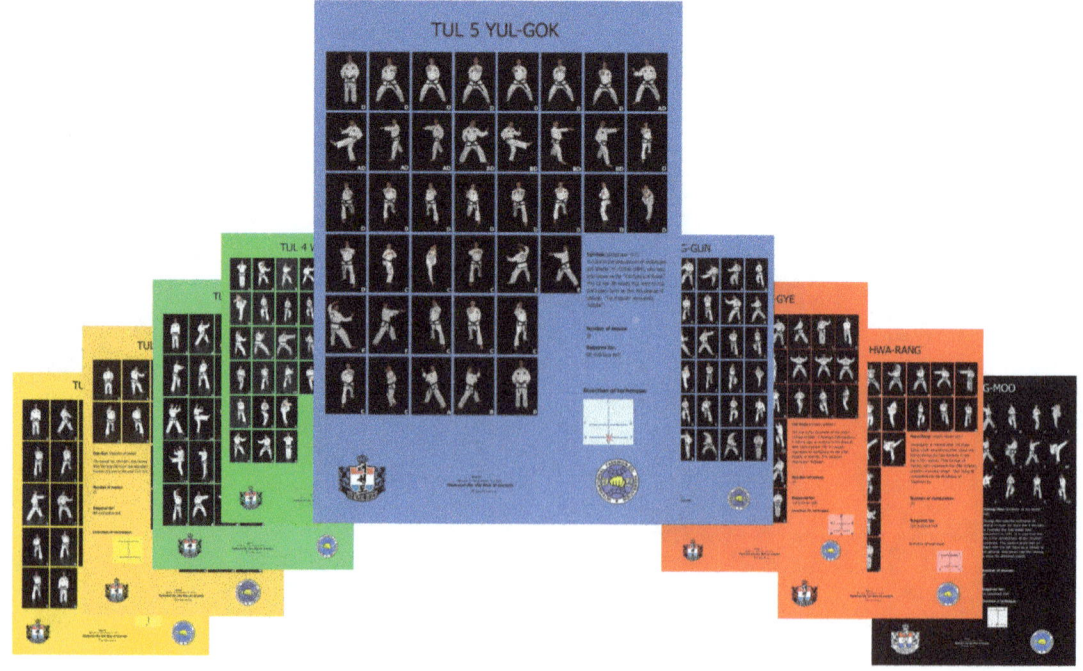

TABLE OF CONTENTS PART 2

PART II – EXERCISE BOOK 11

CHAPTER 1. TAEKWON-DO TECHNIQUES IN PRACTICE 13
1.1 Self-defense against grasping and holding 14
1.2 Tuls in words 21
    Origin 21
    24 tuls 21
    The value of the tul 22
    Starting points of the tuls 24
1.3 Tuls in images 24
    Preparatory tuls 25
    Execution of the tuls 37
     1. Chon-Ji 37
     2. Dan-Gun 46
     3. Do-San 62
     4. Won-Hyo 77
     5. Yul-Gok 93
     6. Joong-Gun 111
     7. Toi-Gye 132
     8. Hwa-Rang 153
     9. Choong-Moo 170
1.4 Step sparring 189
    1-step sparring (*Ilbo-Matsoki*) 193
    2-step sparring (*Ibo-Matsoki*) 193
    Etiquette 194
    1-step sparring set 1 hand technique 195
    1-step sparring set 2 hand technique 199
    1-step sparring set 3 hand technique 201
    1-step sparring set 4 hand technique 203
    1-step sparring set 1 foot technique 207
    1-step sparring set 2 foot technique 209
    1-step sparring set 3 foot technique 211
    2-step sparring set 1 hand technique 215
    2-step sparring set 2 hand technique and front kick 217
    2-step sparring set 3 hand technique and side kick 219
    2-step sparring set 4 hand technique and turning kick 221
    2-step sparring set 5 hand technique and evading/foot technique 223

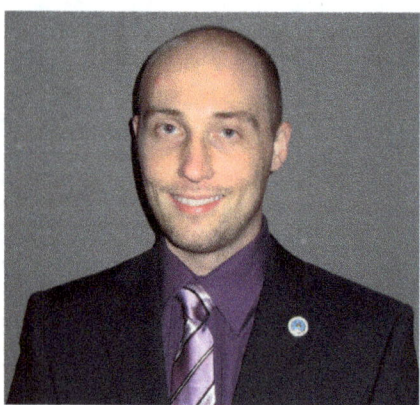

Paul van Beersum
- Internationally acknowledged head teacher
- 4th dan Taekwon-Do (ITF certificate: NED-4-1009)
- 1st dan Hapkido
- International ITF referee A-classification (20-1611)
- Founder and Dojang manager of the Taekwon-Do Academie Gelderland
- Co-founder and board member of ITF Royal Dutch
- Secretary and national coach of the Committee of Technical Education of the ITF Royal Dutch
- Teacher at Taekwon-Do Teacher Training College Committee
- 2nd degree Reiki
- Sports and Movement teacher at Senior Secondary Vocational school ROC A12 in Velp, the Netherlands

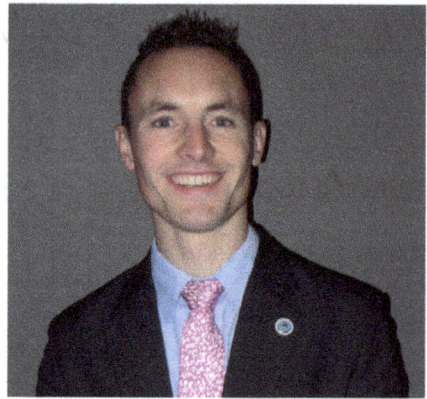

Willem Jansen
- Internationally acknowledged head teacher
- 4th dan Taekwon-Do (ITF certificate: NED-4-1010)
- 1st dan Hapkido
- International ITF referee A-classification (20-1613)
- Founder and Dojang manager of the Taekwon-Do Academie Gelderland
- Co-founder and board member of ITF Royal Dutch
- President and national coach of the Committee of Technical Education of the ITF Royal Dutch
- Teacher at Taekwon-Do Teacher Training College Committee
- Sports masseur
- 1st degree teacher physical education
- President of the physical education department at Olympus College in Arnhem, the Netherlands

www.ingramcontent.com/pod-product-compliance
Lightning Source LLC
Chambersburg PA
CBHW080515110426
42742CB00017B/3120